An Introduction to Performance Analysis of Sport

Performance analysis has become an essential tool for coaches, athletes, sports organisations and academic researchers. Collecting and interpreting performance data enables coaches to improve their training programmes, athletes to make better tactical decisions, sports organisations to manage teams more effectively and researchers to develop a better understanding of sports performance. This fully revised new edition is an essential introduction to the fundamental principles of performance analysis of sport and how to develop and operate performance analysis systems.

Containing worked examples from real sporting events as well as new content examining innovations in determining what to analyse, advances in feedback technology, performance profiles, principles for delivering feedback and telestration within video sequences, *An Introduction to Performance Analysis of Sport* reviews the different types of data and information that performance analysis can generate and explains how to test for reliability.

This cutting-edge book presents a step-by-step guide to developing both manual and computerised analysis systems and writing up and presenting findings from performance analysis programmes. Representing the most up-to-date, concise and engaging introduction to sports performance analysis, this book is an ideal course text for all introductory performance analysis courses, as well as an invaluable primer for coaches and practitioners in sport.

Adam Cullinane is Senior Lecturer in sport performance analysis at Cardiff Metropolitan University and Programme Director of the BSc Sport Performance at the university. He has 12 years' experience in the design and delivery of learning and teaching material within the area of performance analysis. He actively supports students undertaken practical work-based learning. He also contributed heavily to the enterprise initiatives of the Centre for Performance Analysis, where he has provided a range of consultancy services to professional sports teams and NGBs.

Gemma Davies is a Senior Lecturer in sport performance analysis at Cardiff Metropolitan University. She has coupled her academic career with practising as a performance analyst for an NGB, supporting teams at major competitions. This allows her to support students with current applications of analysis from the field. She has experience in leading performance analysis modules and developing learning and teaching material, where she has aligned professional and academic qualifications to enhance a student's portfolio.

Peter O'Donoghue is a professor in sports science at Reykjavik University and general editor of the *International Journal of Performance Analysis in Sport*. He has written, co-authored and edited several books on sports performance analysis and is the editor of the *Routledge Studies in Sports Performance Analysis* series. He has more than 100 peer-reviewed journal publications and has delivered keynote presentations at several world congresses of performance analysis in sport and the world congress of science and racket sports.

Routledge Studies in Sports Performance Analysis

Routledge Studies in Sports Performance Analysis is designed to support students, lecturers and practitioners in all areas of this important and rapidly developing discipline. Books in the series are written by leading international experts in sports performance analysis and cover topics including match analysis, analysis of individual sports and team sports, technique analysis, data analytics, performance analysis for high performance management, and various methodological areas. Drawing on the very latest research, and introducing key concepts and best practice, the series meets a need for accessible, up-to-date texts at all levels of study and work in performance analysis.

Series Editor

Peter O'Donoghue
Reykjavik University

Available in this series:

Performance Analysis in Team Sports
Pedro Passos, Duarte Araújo and Anna Volossovitch

Doing a Research Project in Sport Performance Analysis
Peter O'Donoghue, Lucy Holmes and Gemma Robinson

Professional Practice in Sport Performance Analysis
Edited by Andrew D. Butterworth

An Introduction to Performance Analysis of Sport, Second Edition
Adam Cullinane, Gemma Davies and Peter O'Donoghue

For more information about this series, please visit: https://www.routledge.com/Routledge-Studies-in-Sports-Performance-Analysis/book-series/RSSPA

An Introduction to Performance Analysis of Sport

Second Edition

Adam Cullinane, Gemma Davies and Peter O'Donoghue

Routledge
Taylor & Francis Group
LONDON AND NEW YORK

Designed cover image: Fanatic Studio / Getty

Second edition published 2024
by Routledge
605 Third Avenue, New York, NY 10158

and by Routledge
4 Park Square, Milton Park, Abingdon, Oxon, OX14 4RN

Routledge is an imprint of the Taylor & Francis Group, an informa business

First edition published by Routledge 2015

ISBN: 978-1-032-45115-2 (hbk)
ISBN: 978-1-032-45114-5 (pbk)
ISBN: 978-1-003-37546-3 (ebk)

DOI: 10.4324/9781003375463

Typeset in Bembo
by codeMantra

Adam Cullinane
To my family and friends, thank you for your love and continual support. I would like to express my thanks to all the people who helped me during the writing of this book. In particular, my co-authors Dr Peter O'Donoghue and Gemma Davies, and colleagues in the School of Sport and Health Sciences at Cardiff Metropolitan University.

Gemma Davies
To my family and friends, you have given me the opportunity and time to do what I love. Thank you also to colleagues at Cardiff Metropolitan University and at Wales Netball. It is this partnership that has enabled me to couple life as an academic and applied practitioner, a partnership that has kept me current and armed me with experiences I can forever share with aspiring performance analysts.

Peter O'Donoghue
I made my contributions to this book while working for Cardiff Metropolitan University and Reykjavik University. I wish to dedicate my contributions to my colleagues at both universities. Thank you. Diolch. Takk fyrir.

Contents

Figures

Tables

1 Introduction to sports performance analysis

Introduction

This chapter is roughly divided into two parts. The first part is concerned with sports performance analysis and its purpose within coaching. The first section does touch on other application areas such as uses of performance analysis in the media and officiating. The second part of this chapter is more concerned with the academic discipline of sports performance analysis and discusses research into sports performance and also covers research processes in sports performance analysis as well as writing up sports performance analysis research.

Sports performance analysis in practice

The first edition of this book asked the following questions about sports performance analysis:

- What?
- Why?
- Who?
- When?
- Where?
- How?

This led to different versions of the question "What?" for What is performance analysis? What are the application areas of sports performance analysis? and What information is required? Indeed, when we consider why we do performance analysis, we are also discussing what it is being used for and by whom. So, rather than trying to discuss the what, why, who, when, where and how of sports performance analysis, the second edition of this book will answer a longer list of questions. So, let's begin.

DOI: 10.4324/9781003375463-1

What is sports performance analysis?

Sports performance analysis is primarily a support activity within coaching. Performances are analysed in order to identify areas of good performance as well as areas of performance requiring attention during training. Performances of individuals, teams, opponents and referees can be analysed. The performances can include training as well as match performances. The analysis of performance provides information and valuable insights for coaches and players to support decisions they make about preparation. Performance analysis should not be seen as a threat to players or coaches. Instead, it should be viewed the same way as management information systems are viewed within major businesses and industry. The information is produced for use by the coaches and players, and it is very much a service in this respect to allow more informed decisions to be made.

Why do we analyse sports performance?

As mentioned above, performance analysis produces information to inform coaching decisions. However, the rationale for performance analysis support comes from the knowledge of coach recall in the absence of such information. Detailed recollection of events is difficult in many areas of life. Studies of eye-witness testimony have highlighted limitations in the ability of humans to accurately recall events (Benton et al., 2006; Bornstein, 2017; Loftus, 2019; Wixted and Wells, 2017). I want you to think about somebody you met and spoke to today. What were they wearing? What colour were their shoes? What colours were the other items of clothing they were wearing? There is nothing unusual about struggling to remember such details, even when it is important to remember such details. We are very efficient in our use of information in our daily lives, that we sometimes only recall what we really need to recall to do what we need to do or get where we need to go? Now I want you to think of somewhere you travelled in recent days, perhaps shopping, or to work or college, or to your home. Think about some landmarks on the journey that you must have passed on the route you took. Can you remember passing these landmarks on this particular journey? Can you remember what was happening at these landmarks? Can you remember whether it was busy with people or quiet at the different landmarks? Again, if you are struggling to recall some of this information, there is nothing unusual about this. This also applies in coaching. An early study by Franks and Miller (1986) found that novice coaches only accurately recall 42% of critical incidents from matches on average. They also found that the accuracy of recall varied between different events, with details of set pieces being recalled more accurately than details of other events. Laird and Waters (2008) did a similar study finding that 59% of critical incidents were accurately recalled by qualified soccer coaches. This improvement may be due to the more qualified coaches used in Laird and Waters' (2008) study and advances made in continuous professional development for coaches since the 1980s. While there has been improvement between 1986 and 2008, coaches still have an incomplete and inaccurate recollection of the match. There are a number of reasons for this, including bias and favouritism influencing coaches' perceptions of events. Fatigue may also play a role in coaches' ability to concentrate during the match. They may be distracted from key events during the match if their attention is focused on other areas. This is understandable, especially in team sports where it is not possible to observe all of the players all of the time. Simply looking down to write something in a notebook can cause a coach to miss something important that occurs. A further reason for inaccurate recall of events is emotional involvement in the game. This can be experienced by spectators as well as the coaches and players involved. While the outcome of a contest may be uncertain, viewers may consider the chance of a successful outcome to be lower than it actually is. The first edition of this book described the author's perceptions of a professional boxing match he was watching live at the venue. The author felt that the boxer he was supporting was losing the contest up until the point when he won on a stoppage. Subsequently, the author was able to view a video recording of the contest in full knowledge of the result and, on this occasion, he felt the boxer was leading on points from the end of the first round. Readers will probably be able to compare their own perceptions of sports contests they have watched both live and on video afterwards. Timing of feedback can also impact the accuracy of recall. For example, Jones et al. (2004) suggested that the accuracy of recall decreases over time and that delays in providing feedback may result in inaccurate feedback being provided. Given the misperceptions of performance that can result from bias, emotion, fatigue and the limited ability of humans to remember detail, there is a strong rationale for having an accurate record of a sports contest. This can take the form of video recording, match statistics or a combination of both.

Who uses the sports performance information?

The previous subsection of this chapter concentrated on coach and player use of the information generated by performance analysis. The information is also of use to other management and support staff in the coaching context. High-performance managers can use the information from multiple matches to identify trends and make strategic decisions that are at a higher level than day-to-day coaching decisions. Performance analysts can also provide information to other members of the sports science support staff. For example, performance analysts may work closely with strength and conditioning coaches, helping them analyse movement data. This may be data from GPS devices or other player tracking technology. There have also been examples where sports psychologists have requested video sequences of periods of play they wish to discuss with the squad or individual players. It is typically the performance analyst who deals with the match videos and who may do some ad hoc analyses of these videos to provide the necessary sequences to the sports psychologist. Some large performance analysis departments within professional clubs may have "recruitment analysts" who may liaise with scouts as well as coaches. A detailed discussion of performance analysis within multidisciplinary teams and interdisciplinary teams can be found in Butterworth's book (2023b). The distinction between multidisciplinary and interdisciplinary approaches is where collaboration between sports science support services happens. Within multidisciplinary approaches, these services tackle common problems and eventually discuss the problem from their different perspectives. By contrast, the collaboration between sports science support services commences from the outset of dealing with a problem in an interdisciplinary approach. This chapter of Butterworth's book describes the types of problems in sport that benefit from an integrated use of performance analysis and other sports science support services. It also recognises the barriers that exist to multidisciplinary and interdisciplinary sports science support as well as the importance of establishing frameworks to manage integrated sports science support. The integrated use of information streams from multiple sports science support services is also important in the strategic management of high-performance sport (Wiltshire, 2013). Wiltshire describes how high-performance management systems should be holistic covering physical, psychological, medical, performance lifestyle as well as the technical and tactical information used in coaching.

Besides the use of sports performance information within coaching, there are other uses of the information. There are broadcast and media uses of match statistics to help commentators and enhance the viewer experience by providing additional talking points. Kirkbride (2013) used the term "infotainment" to cover the broad spectrum of performance analysis activity within broadcast coverage of sport as well as social media. In recent years, there has been an increase in the availability of data about sports events targeting the betting market. Apps providing such data rely on data being collected using special purpose systems live during matches. Thus, we can see coders working live at matches using special purpose data entry systems. The authors have personally met students they have taught who collect data for these platforms. The need for reliable coders has meant that some have been recruited before completing their undergraduate degrees and they code matches as a weekend job. Sometimes, an analyst may be recording more than one match per day where the matches commence at different times but in the same general locality. Sports performance data can also be analysed by those concerned with "sports integrity". Data analysis, in itself, cannot prove that match fixing, for example, has occurred, but it can alert interested parties to where it may have occurred. Omoigui (2022) interviewed Jake Marsh, the global head of integrity at StatsPerform (Stats Perform Group, Chicago, IL) about the range of work they do including monitoring of sports performance and the integrated analysis of performance data and betting patterns. A challenge for detecting match fixing is that the performances of teams and individual players vary. Indeed, variability in sports performance has been an important area of research over the last 20 years (Bliss et al., 2022; Gregson et al., 2010; Hopkins and Hewson, 2001; Malcata and Hopkins, 2014). Therefore, there is a need to understand normal variability in sports performance in order to be able to detect potentially abnormal performances. This can be quite sophisticated given that some performers may be more consistent than others. An example of this was Henry Stott's predictive modelling of the 2002 FIFA (Fédération Internationale de Football Association) men's World Cup where he found that the opening match between France and Senegal was one of the five matches most likely to be an upset. An upset was counted as a match where a team lost against a lower ranked team according to the FIFA World rankings (Mayfield, 2022). This match was actually an upset with Senegal winning 1–0. Stott included "patchiness" (or inconsistency) of teams' performances within his model. This meant that a match between two relatively inconsistent teams could be more likely to be an upset than a match between two more consistent teams who were closer to each other in the FIFA World rankings. UEFA (Union of European Football Associations) are conducting research into variability in soccer performance in collaboration with Middlesex University (Parmar, 2023). Specifically, they are profiling performance to analyse "change in performance". Whether or not this is to be applied in the detection of match fixing is unknown by the author of this chapter at the time of writing, but it would be a potential application area.

Those who judge sports performances would not consider themselves to be performance analysts. Certainly, referees and umpires have a different role to performance analysts. They observe contests in order to apply the rules rather than discover useful insights for the performers. Nonetheless, there are activities within the officiating of sports contests that are similar to what performance analysts do in coaching scenarios. One only has to think of some of the images shown of VAR (Video Assisted Refereeing) rooms during the 2022 FIFA men's World Cup to appreciate the use of technology to review play for this purpose. The criteria used to assess sports like trampoline, gymnastics, diving and figure skating require judges to analyse performance in a similar level of detail to analysts working with athletes and coaches. This subsection is more concerned with analysis of referee, umpire and judge performance rather than the observational analysis activity of the officials themselves. Governing bodies in sport can monitor referee performance and give feedback to them after matches. Research has found gymnastics judging to be sufficiently valid and reliable (Bučar et al., 2012; Pizzera et al., 2018), while research into diving scoring has been evaluated against performance variables determined from video observation (Luedeker and McKee, 2023). Johns and Bourner (2013) compared trampoline judge performance with an observational approach applying scoring criteria to lapse-time video observation. Statistics on refereeing performance are now provided for some sports (Whoscored, 2023) and may be useful to teams playing in matches where the referees are in charge. Performance analysis research has considered the accuracy of refereeing decisions in team games (García-Santos et al., 2020) as well as the physical demands of refereeing (Blair et al., 2022). Physical demands can be analysed using a combination of distance, speed and heart rate variables (Bester et al., 2019). Some research has investigated the decision making of officials in team games, considering their positioning on the field of play (Lima e Silva et al., 2020; SantaAnna et al., 2021). SantaAnna et al. (2021) concluded that referees may move in energy efficient ways during the second half of matches. Observational analysis of referee behaviour during matches also permits communicative behaviours and interaction with players to be investigated (Lewis et al., 2023). Another area of interest is the additional time awarded by referees in soccer and how this relates to relevant stoppages that occurred during matches (Prüßner and Siegle, 2015).

Coach behaviour can also be analysed during coaching qualifications or continuous professional development (Franks et al., 2001). There are systems, such as the Arizona State University Observation Instrument (Lacy and Darst, 1989), that have been used in research but which can also be used to provide feedback to coaches about their use of demonstrations, silent monitoring, instruction and other behaviours during coaching. The set of behaviours used in the Arizona State University Observation Instrument is relatively simple and the system does not include additional descriptor information about the context of the behaviours or audience for communication events. Cushion (2018) discussed some of the complexities of coach behaviour that can be addressed by those seeking to use observational analysis within coach development programmes. Coach behaviour analysis systems have been used to tag coach behaviour allowing interactive viewing of coach behaviour to help coaches reflect on their coaching style (Brown and O'Donoghue, 2008). Figure 1.1 is an example of such a system.

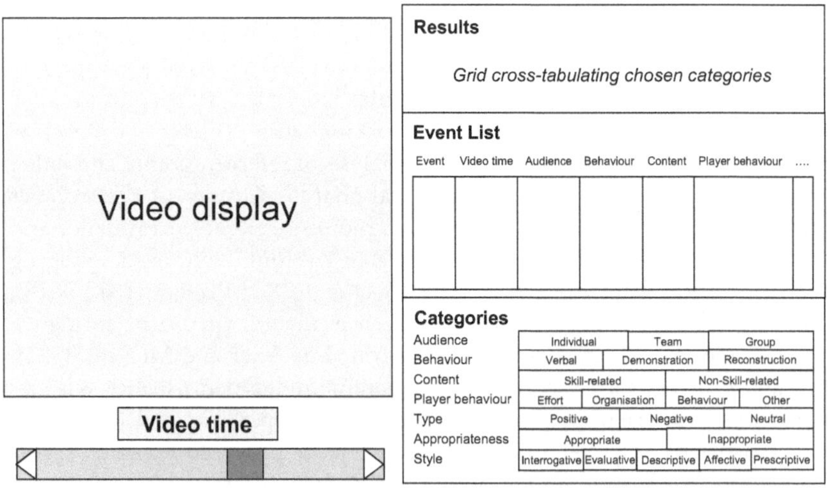

Figure 1.1 Analysing coaching behaviour using Focus X2.

Who analyses the performances?

The obvious answer to this question is that performance analysts analyse performances and produce information for coaches, players and other users. There are performance analysts who are employed directly by sports squads and governing bodies. Some of these analysts may have specialist roles within analysis departments. For example, recent job adverts in professional soccer have included "recruitment analyst", "set piece analyst", "opposition analyst", "individual development coach/analyst", "video scout", "academy analyst", "coach analyst", "lead analyst", "head of performance analysis" and "assistant analyst". An inspection of the Twitter account of the Association of Professional Football Analysts (APFA, n.d.) gives an indication of how frequently such positions are advertised. These positions are typically for specific squads or age groups.

Some squads may have links with universities allowing students to gain work experience as performance analysts. Academic credit can be accumulated for such work where university programmes have placement or work-experience elements. There are clear benefits for students taking on such placements but also concerns about potential exploitation of unpaid interns (Butterworth, 2023d; Butterworth and O'Donoghue, 2023). Butterworth (2023d) describes the importance of having experience in sports performance analysis when applying for professional roles in the area. Developing technical skills, intellectual ability and academic knowledge about sports performance are all important. However, an applicant for a professional analyst role who has demonstrated that they can gather valid data using reliable methods and provide statistical and video sequence feedback in an efficient manner will have an edge over applicants with no such experience. Thus, most performance analysis programmes now include work experience modules.

There are freelance analysts who may work with squads in a number of sports as well as teach part-time in college or university. Where squads use the services of freelance analysts, they have the advantage of not needing to purchase the analysis software or hardware needed. It may help if a squad working with a freelance analyst does have its own copies of the analysis software so that coaches and players can interactively view and discuss video sequences that the analyst has tagged. Indeed, there are coaches who are well skilled at using the software systems for review tasks. Where squads don't have copies of the software systems, video sequences can be shared using normal file sharing processes or the squads may elect to use coach information management packages such as CoachLogic (CoachLogic, Edinburgh, UK) or My Team Performance (My Team Performance, Hertogenbosch, Netherlands) to share video sequences with players.

It has already been mentioned that some coaches operate match analysis software themselves when reviewing performances. This is typically after an analyst has tagged the match and provided the match statistics and key take home messages. There are some coaches who analyse matches without the use of an analyst (Martin et al., 2018). This is typically due to budget constraints, but where the coach is still keen to use performance information to help players develop. Players have also been provided with facilities to tag elements of their own performances (Flick, 2016). This process of tagging videos of performances can help players recognise areas of the game where they can improve and facilitate discussions with other players and coaches. This also gives them control of the quantity, timing, pace and content of the feedback.

Sports performances are also analysed by analysis companies that serve multiple squads in the same sport. This type of analysis is a much larger scale operation than what is done by freelance analysts. Freelance analysts might not be able to work with more than one squad in a single competition due to their knowledge of discussions with coaches and players. Larger scale analysis companies, like StatsPerform, who provide Opta data to multiple sports (Stats Perform Group, Chicago, Il), and Statsbomb (StatsBomb Inc., Bath, UK), are able to provide data services to multiple squads within the same competitions because their analysts do not work directly with the squads. The analysis that is done is typically using standard variables, in some cases allowing all teams in a competition to use data from all of the matches in the competition, not just the matches the teams participate in.

Where? And when?

Another "What?" question ("What is sports performance analysis research?") is deferred until the second part of this chapter. A further question is "What should be analysed?" which is the subject of Chapter 3 of the current book. How to do the analysis has been touched upon when answering some of the questions asked so far. However, more detail of manual and computerised methods is provided in Chapters 4–7. This leaves us considering the where and the when of sports performance analysis activities. Once performance analysis systems have been developed and are in operation, the main activities of performance analysis can be broadly grouped into data collection, data analysis and communication of information. The classic coaching process models of Franks (1997) for analysing broad tactical and technical events in game sports and Irwin et al. (2013) for more detailed analysis of technique intensive sports show these activities performed in a cycle. Figure 1.2 shows Frank's (1997) model where the performance analysis activities typically occur between matches. Thus, the game is played, performance data are collected live or post-match, analysed and then feedback takes place informing preparation for the next match. In Irwin et al.'s (2013) model, analysis activities are performed in a cycle between performances which could be training or competitive performances. Thus, developing technique is monitored over time through data collection and analysis. Advances in technology have permitted highly efficient data gathering and data processing allowing live

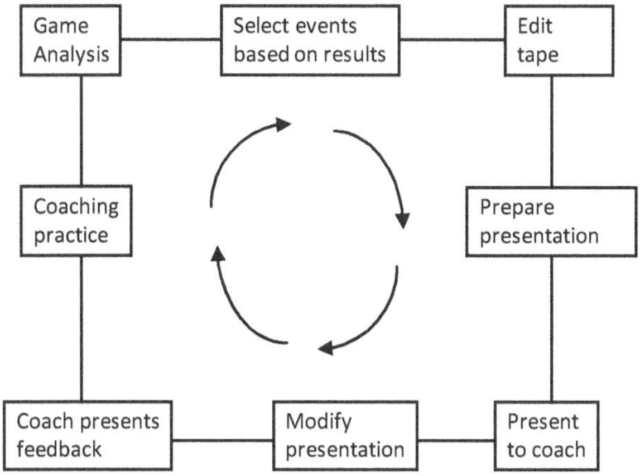

Figure 1.2 Frank's (1997) coaching process.

feedback to be provided during competition (Jayal et al., 2018: 18–20). The concurrent provision of information to coaches and players during competition, while data are still being gathered and analysed, is a characteristic of the analytics era. An example of such a process can be observed during television coverage of Formula One motor racing where in-race decision making is informed by simulation of tactical options requiring large volumes of data and high-performance computer processing. These processes require such levels of flexibility, staff expertise and multiple data streams that they cannot be represented by traditional models of performance analysis in coaching.

The locations where sports performance activities occur are similar to those described in O'Donoghue's (2010) first book. Where data are collected live during competitions, this can be done at the competition venue or away from the competition venue if the performance is being displayed live on television or through web-streaming. The use of IP cameras allows data to be collected from anywhere with internet access. There are occasions where match events can be recorded using a palm-top computer and then the event list can be synchronised with a video of the match later. There are also situations where some data are collected live during competition while other data are added post-match. Technological advances allow more data to be gathered during matches. An example of this is where additional analysts can enter data on iPad devices and these events are sent to the main analyst's computer and added to the main timeline. This not only allows for more data to be gathered live during the match but also means that more data can be entered at the venue before the team depart after the match.

Once data have been collected, they can be analysed. The fact that events have been tagged and are stored on computer disk permits very efficient processing using the features of the video analysis package. These features include matrices allowing events to be cross-tabulated with descriptor values. These matrices or the raw event lists can be exported for further analysis in packages such as Microsoft Excel (Microsoft, Redmond, WA). Spreadsheets can be programmed to process the exported data meaning that the same spreadsheet template can be used with multiple matches, making data analysis particularly efficient. This analysis is typically quantitative, determining frequencies and percentage conversion rates, possibly classifying the resulting values based on norms for the given level of competition. Decisions need to be made about video sequences to use within feedback to players. This is a different process to the preceding quantitative analyses of tagged events. Analysts and coaches need to decide on the video sequences using expert knowledge of the sport. Telestration tools can be used to highlight important areas of key video frames. These analysis activities can be done at a variety of locations including the match venue, the analyst's office, a performance analysis laboratory, hotel room, the analyst's home or anywhere else a computer can be operated.

Once data have been analysed, the resulting statistics and video sequences can be presented. This can be done collectively or individually. Internet-based coaching management systems such as CoachLogic and My Team Performance allow players to engage with the information at times and locations that suit them. This allows online discussions to take place before players meet at training sessions. The importance of this is that it allows more time for actual training when players do meet up. Communications technologies used in social media are very familiar to players today and can be used for sharing information, again supporting more flexible and convenient feedback to players. Thus, players can engage with feedback anywhere where they can use their own devices that support the communications platforms being used.

Sports performance analysis research

What is research?

This second part of this chapter discusses sports performance research rather than performance analysis in the coaching context. Before getting into sports performance research, it is worth briefly introducing research in general. Research can be performed in many different contexts and in many different ways. Research can be done by lawyers or detectives investigating cases, journalists, industrial research and development departments, market research for commercial organisations or by academics studying their fields of interest. Research can be applied to a direct real-world problem or it can be purely to generate knowledge without a direct real-world application at the time of the study. This range of research studies has been described as a "continuum" by some authors of research methods textbooks (Thomas and Nelson, 1996: 5–7). Research can be considered in terms of communication, evidence and quality.

Communication is an essential stage of research. When a study is completed, the authors should communicate their findings so that the knowledge can be used by others and we continue to learn. Consider the fact that we live in buildings with running water, sanitation, electricity, furniture, and heating. All of this is possible because of discoveries being made over time, communicated, exploited, integrated with other knowledge and applied. It is not possible for any one person to make all of the discoveries that we benefit from in our everyday lives. So, researchers often work in niche areas using existing knowledge as a starting point for their own research. The communication of knowledge to others takes many forms, for example, articles in scientific research journals, technical reports within organisations as well as oral or poster presentations at conferences. It is this ability to communicate that makes what we have discovered available to others, and a reason why we live more comfortable lives than other species who do not have human communication skills. Publicly funded research comes with a duty to publish. This has led to some tensions from what is referred to as the "open access" era. Completing and publishing research does not come for free because people's time is not free. Those undertaking the research as well as staff within the publishing companies who produce scientific journals all perform activities that have costs. On the one hand, there is a view that publicly funded research should be freely available rather than behind the "pay wall" of a commercial publisher's journal. There would be some merit to this argument if the public funding fully covered all publication costs as well as the research itself, but this is rarely the case. The other side of the argument is that there must be some incentive to doing research in order to encourage research to continue. Piracy has been a problem with research material, that some access as paying subscribers to journals, being made freely and illegally available to others. Other tensions arise from research audits that inform funding decisions for university research. Specifically, for papers to be included in national research audits, they often have to be made available on university research repositories. The availability of research articles in such repositories can make some universities question whether they need to subscribe to certain journals.

The previous paragraph was getting increasingly controversial, so we will turn to evidence. Research should be a systematic process of studying the subject of interest, gathering and analysis data and drawing conclusions that are supported by the data. This is in contrast to non-scientific ways of generating knowledge such as intuition, speculation and hunches (Martens, 1987). Those using research should not blindly accept the findings of studies but should consider how the research was done and whether studies have limitations. This would be the same with any other evidence trail from which conclusions are being drawn. Readers of research studies should be critical and question the variables that were used, when the data were collected, how the data were collected, who participated in the study and how the data were analysed. Research should be rigorous and transparent if it is to contribute to knowledge. Valid and relevant variables should be used, data should be gathered and analysed using trustworthy and reliable processes. There is also something for scholars to consider when they refer to research in their own studies. The evidence of a research study comes from what was found and how the study was done. Scholars should not be referring to a paper as evidence of a comment made in the introduction section of the paper or the discussion. These comments are more speculation and discussion points rather than the real evidence provided by the paper. It is fair to say that much of what has been discussed here is about empirical research and the authors of the current book recognise the value of other types of research including philosophical research.

The previous paragraph about research evidence has already covered some elements of research quality. Research quality can be judged on originality, rigour and impact. Originality is an interesting research quality to discuss. Where a study is essentially repeating a study that has already been done, but perhaps with different participants, it may not be contributing new knowledge. However, there is a role for studies to confirm or refute the findings of previous studies based on the conclusions drawn from the data. As sport develops, it is important to keep research up-to-date because of rule changes and other developments. It may be necessary for a study to be repeated with a larger sample, involving multiple countries, in order to give the necessary confidence for policy makers to consider the findings of the research. Findings of research which may have been done in one level, or age group, or gender might not be generalisable beyond these groups prompting the need for further research which is not entirely original, but nonetheless needed.

Rigour is to do with the care that has been taken in gathering and analysing data for a research study. Some variables can be measured more accurately than others; this is sometimes aided by the use of precise measuring equipment. Validity is the first measurement issue to be considered. A hyper-accurate variable is not going to be of interest to readers if it is a "so what?" or "who cares?" variable. However, a clearly relevant variable that cannot be reliably measured can be considered invalid if the values recorded are compromised by subjective data collection processes. An example of a validity to reliability trade-off is the number of forced and unforced errors made in tennis performances. Errors can be distinguished from winners relatively easily and with a high level of reliability. If a ball lands in the opponent's court and cannot be played by the opponent before it bounces for a second time, then the shot is a winner. If the ball lands outside the opponent's court or strikes the net, failing to make the opponent's court, then the shot is an error. Distinguishing between forced and unforced errors is more difficult and requires knowledge of the sport by those gathering the data. Counts of unforced errors are of interest to practitioners and are also provided in media coverage of tennis matches. However, when a shot is returning a previous shot that is well placed, with high velocity and played with spin, it can be difficult to class an error as an unforced error, especially at elite levels of the sport.

The impact of research is concerned with its real-world application. Real-world benefit of research has become more important in recent years. An example of this is the UK Research Excellence Framework (REF) requiring impact case studies for universities to make submissions in different subject areas. While research can be argued to have real-world benefit, it is often difficult to evidence that research has informed policies or practices in the real-world. Hence, the impact case studies submitted to the REF show where research has been used, how it has been used, by whom and with evidence of any benefits. This requires minutes of meetings or other evidence showing that real-world action was supported by the research that had been done.

To complete this general section on research, it is worth considering the quality of research that is necessary for publication in a scientific journal. Shore (1991) listed seven sources of scientific dishonesty, one of which was non-publication of data. Shore was specifically talking about situations where dishonest researchers may remove data from a study so that the remaining data supports some conclusion they wish to make. There are valid reasons for excluding data from studies and these reasons are stated within the methods sections of research articles. For example, one might not wish to include matches where players have been dismissed from studies of team game performance. The exclusion of data referred to by Shore (1991) is a different type of removal of data and should not be done. This leads to a wider question of whether a study that has been completed and written up in a transparent manner should ever be rejected. Rejecting such a paper is essentially non-publication of data on a larger scale, concealing the paper from the public as though the study does not exist. There has been speculation that papers where effects or relationships are found to be statistically significant are more likely to be published than papers where analysis of the data has not produced statistically significant results (Schmucker et al., 2014). However, any bias towards publication of studies with significant results could be due to researchers not submitting papers where the results were not significant (Dickerson et al., 1992). Publication policies in sports performance analysis are illustrated by the 646 papers submitted to the International Journal of Performance Analysis in Sport in the calendar year 2022. Only 46 of these papers were actually published, suggesting 13 papers are rejected for every paper that is selected. However, there are papers rejected from the journal because they are not sports performance analysis papers, outside the scope of the journal, and that needed to be sent elsewhere. The remaining papers were ultimately rejected for the following reasons:

- The results were achieved through a misuse of statistics, for example, treating events from a small number of matches as though they are independent.
- The reliability of the variables used has not been established.
- Data have been gathered from secondary sources, such as internet sites, in violation of the terms of use of these data sources.
- Data have come from a single squad, possibly a convenience sample, and possibly collected for reasons other than research, and cannot be generalised beyond the squad.

- Lack of transparency in the description methods.
- Lack of impact where the study is too specific to be of general interest to the journal's subscribers,
- The data are out of date and there may have been substantial rule changes in the sport since the data were collected.
- The research work may not represent a substantial research effort and could be done in a weekend.
- Misinterpretation of data and apparent lack of knowledge of research in the area based on the discussion section.
- Poor scientific writing, including lack of supporting references for arguments made in the introduction and discussion.

Some of these reasons are straightforward, but others are worth further consideration. Should single squad studies ever be published? Yes! There is a serious need for evidence that feedback based on sports performance data has an impact in coaching. In-depth case studies about experiences of using performance analysis in sport are time consuming, complex and with ethical issues to be addressed. These difficulties are one reason for so few case studies being published or even being attempted.

Consider a study that has been done efficiently in a short amount of time, using data with proper permissions, from a secondary source, with evidence provided that the secondary data are valid and reliable. The decision for the paper to be published or not needs to consider the originality and need for the study, the novelty of the analysis of the data, theoretical development and interest in the paper. Thus, publishing such a paper is not ruled out. However, the research community needs to be mindful of standards set for journal publication, especially when there are other outlets for presenting smaller scale research. The kind of thing that can be problematic is where a researcher conducts four such studies, without having to make the efforts other researchers need to in order to gather data. It is highly questionable whether such a programme of research is substantive enough to be awarded a doctorate, yet publishing this number of papers from postgraduate research would typically be seen as evidence of doctoral level research. In the UK, a doctorate would be the equivalent of three years of level 8 research work; this is 540 credit points or 5,400 effort hours of work at this level. So, we are looking for thousands of hours of research activity rather than tens of hours of research activity for a research project to be considered substantial enough for journal publication.

One of the reasons given for rejecting a paper was "lack of impact". An example of this is where research teams are undertaking a programme of research in an area that may well be very interesting and worthwhile. However, they attempt to get the reliability study of their analysis system published as a journal article. The issue here is that the system is a very specific system that might only ever be used in their programme of research. An editor's response to this might be to use the system to do a research study and incorporate the certification of reliability into the methods section of that paper. Typically, the authors have intended to use the system for useful and interesting research, but are attempting to "salami slice" a paper into more than one paper. Indeed, some authors also attempt to publish the background section of a research paper as a separate paper calling it a "systematic review". There is a place for systematic reviews in well-developed areas of research. However, some systematic reviews submitted to the International Journal of Performance Analysis of Sport have been in very narrow areas or areas where research has not developed sufficiently to justify a review article.

The penultimate bullet point seems to contradict an earlier point in this chapter where we stated the real evidence of a study comes from what was found and the methods used in the research. The type of thing that research journals need to avoid is where somebody from an unconnected field, who is lacking in knowledge of the field of interest to the journal, is able to analyse some data and produce results to answer some question because they are good at statistics. Imagine, for example, someone comparing tennis matches played on different court surfaces, not knowing that different ball types are used on different court surfaces, and drawing inappropriate conclusions about a surface effect. This would be a good reason to reject the paper.

What are the purposes of sports performance analysis research?

Sports performance analysis is an area of sports science where actual sports performance is being investigated. This could be performance during competition or training, or possibly performance of game related skills under more controlled conditions. Examples of the latter are where things like the serve in tennis or a golf swing are analysed in laboratory experiments. While this is not actual sports performance, the actions being performed are key parts of the sports and it may not be feasible to collect detailed data about technique during actual sports performance. The kind of research that would normally not qualify as sports performance analysis research are analyses of fitness tests, interview and questionnaires. The issue with performing fitness tests is that the tests and measurements are not actual sports performance. It is possible that test results might be correlated with variables from actual sports performance. The variables derived from actual sports performance need to represent enough performance analysis research for the study to be considered within the scope of a performance analysis journal. Interviews and questionnaires are useful for gathering data from participants about their attitudes and beliefs. However, sports performance analysis is about what players actually do rather than what they report that they do. In saying this, there are occasions where survey research makes welcome contribution to sports performance theory. Later in this section, we will discuss research into the effectiveness of performance analysis support in coaching. Such studies use interviews and questionnaires in the investigation of coach and player attitude towards and use of performance analysis services.

The main purposes of sports performance analysis research are in the areas of technical effectiveness, tactics, physical demands of sports and effectiveness of performance analysis support services. The first three types of study can be done in a descriptive way where independent variables are hypothesised to have an influence on dependent variables which may be about the skills performed, tactics or physical demands. Starting with the dependent variables, technical effectiveness can be distinguished from more detailed analysis of technique. In technical effectiveness, we simply record that players performed skills like passes, shots, forehand strokes, backhand strokes, etc. and whether those skills were performed successfully or not. These data are then used to determine variables such as the frequency of techniques of different types as well as the percentage of applications of each technique that are performed successfully. Examples of such studies are Timmons et al.'s (2022) study of kickouts in Gaelic football and Liu et al.'s (2022) study of strokes in table tennis.

Tactical analysis tends to analyse the same skills as when we are analysing technical effectiveness. However, tactical analysis is more concerned with what teams do than how well they do it. The profile of skills performed is often not enough to indicate tactics, and so additional information about the pitch locations where skills are performed, timings and players involved can also give an indication of tactical decisions. Ultimately tactical decisions are made by players during games, considering the options they have and the relative advantages and disadvantages of these. Such decisions are not directly observable to researchers, but inferences can be made about these decisions using information about what players ultimately do in different situations. Tactical analysis can be applied to broader passages of play rather than individual skills that are performed. Examples are possessions of the ball in team games where the locations and timings of individual skills can indicate that particular tactics have been chosen. While tactical analysis is more about what has been done rather than how well it has been done, there are many studies that have also looked at how well alternative tactics are performed based on success rates. Examples of research into tactics include O'Donoghue and Beckley's (2023) study of possessions in the Euro 2022 soccer tournament and Laxdal et al.'s (2022) study of Icelandic league handball.

Decision making is related to tactics but there is a subtle difference between performance analysis research into decision making. In tactical analysis, we are ultimately investigating the chosen tactics that are represented by observable behaviour. Analysis of decision making goes beyond this to also consider the quality of decision making. Specifically, the analysis of decision making not only analyses decisions made, but considers decisions that could have been made (Lorains et al., 2013; Parrington et al., 2013). In netball, expert players have more options available to them when passing than novice players do (Bruce et al., 2009). In order to draw this conclusion, it was necessary for Bruce et al. (2009) to analyse video frames for each pass in their study and assess the number of realistic options the passing player had. The number of options open to players has also been investigated in Australian rules football (Parrington et al., 2013). A further study of Australian rules football classified the quality of each decision as "best", "good", "last" or "bad" (Lorains et al., 2013). The analysis of number of options and quality of decision made goes beyond what typical tactical analysis studies do. Mobile eye tracking equipment has been used to investigate eye fixations during experimental vide decision making tasks with occlusion of scenes 120 ms before the player in the video performed an action (Vítor de Assis et al, 2020). This analysis was combined with decision accuracy scores revealing that higher skilled players required less fixation time and made more accurate decisions.

The demands of a game can be characterised by the profile of skills that players of different positional roles perform. The physical demands of a sport, on the other hand, are evaluated using movement data, particularly considering periods of high speed running and recovery between these. Accelerations, decelerations, impacts, jumps and turns can also be included in the data analysed about physical demands (Bloomfield et al., 2004; Rayner et al., 2022) with other studies incorporating heart rate data recorded during matches (Roldán-Márquez et al., 2022). Examples of research into the physical demands of sports include Kádár et al.'s (2023) study of Hungarian soccer players at different age groups and Gong et al.'s (2021) study of Chinese Super League soccer that combined physical and technical variables.

The independent variables for studies into tactics, technical effectiveness of physical demands can be grouping variables like age group, gender, playing position or competition type. Alternatively, they may be situational variables (Gómez et al., 2013) such as venue, match status (score-line), opposition quality or numerical superiority. Some studies compare winning and losing teams to identify performance indicators associated with match outcome (García-Marín and Iturriaga, 2017). The outcome of a match can be seen as being more of a dependent variable than an independent variable. This had led some researchers to use predictive models to associate game outcome with process indicators (Koo et al., 2016).

There is overlap between sports performance analysis and other disciplines of sports science. This is because when we are analysing sports performance, we are analysing some aspect of sports performance such as work rate or tactical movement. When we investigate work rate in team games, we typically discuss intermittent high intensity activity, referring to physiology research that has investigated energy systems used in intermittent high intensity activity. When we analyse momentum or score-line effects, we would discuss findings in relation to sports psychology. Analysing technique is related to biomechanics, and other sports performance analysis research is discussed using material from coaching science and strength and conditioning.

The fourth purpose of research into sports performance analysis is to evaluate performance analysis services in coaching contexts. This can be done by interviewing coaches (Anderson et al., 2021), interviewing athletes (Fernandez-Echeverria et al., 2019; Loo et al., 2020), interviewing analysts

(Martin et al., 2021) or analysing trends in performance for a squad along with in-depth qualitative data about the role of performance analysis and feedback in achieving results. A study of martial arts used interviews with six coaches and six boxers to explore the role of performance analysis technology within debriefings and the wider issues of feedback and communication in the coaching environment (Kojman et al., 2022). An example of an in-depth study of performance analysis support in coaching is Butterworth's (2023a; 2023c) work with an international netball squad. Huggan et al. (2015) used a story telling approach to present the findings of a series of interviews they did with a soccer analyst to characterise the micropolitical environment of performance analysis in soccer in a way that protected the identity of the participant and club involved in the study.

Writing up sports performance research

As with other areas of sports science, there are a variety of ways of communicating research that has been done using sports performance analysis methods. Writing commences before data collection commences as studies need to be planned and approved. Research proposals are done by undergraduate students, taught postgraduate students, postgraduate researchers as well as senior researchers in educational establishments and research institutes. The research proposal typically contains a background to the research problem, articulates a need for the research, states the objectives and describes the research design and methods (Kumar, 2005: 188–189). It may also include a timetable of activity that will occur during the research project. The methods are written in the future tense. This may seem like an obvious thing to say, but many students do make the mistake of writing the methods section of a research proposal in the past tense when they are describing research that is going to be done in the future. Student research proposals are scrutinised to ensure the project involves an appropriate volume of research and is feasible, relevant to their programme of study and ethical. Research proposals are also done by senior researchers applying for research grants. These proposals have additional contents about staff, equipment, consumable and travel costs.

Writing up a research project typically commences before the research is completed. For example, students can complete introduction and literature review sections before data collection commences. Data collection and write-up activity can run in parallel. Parts of the methods chapter can be written before data collection is completed. Once a system has been developed, tested for reliability and used for some data collection, the student will be able to start the methods chapter. Essentially, they will be writing about what they have been doing. The methods chapters of performance analysis dissertations may be longer than methods chapters in other areas of sports science because many performance analysis projects are using new variables and cannot simply refer to existing material to describe data collection and analysis. The methods chapter of a sports performance analysis dissertation typically contains sections on research design, system development, reliability evaluation, matches, data collection and data analysis. The section on system development should include descriptions of the variables being used and pilot work during system development. There is usually a single results chapter within a dissertation that includes all of the findings whether quantitative or qualitative. In quantitative research, summary results should be presented using tables, charts as well as possibly including pitch diagrams if location of events are important. Where qualitative research has been done the findings may be integrated with the discussion rather than separating these chapters. Qualitative findings can include exerts of raw interview data (quotes) that characterise the findings. The discussion chapter explains the results and discusses the findings in the light of existing published research. The discussion should be organised into broad areas that can be discussed holistically rather than using a result by result approach. The conclusions chapter sums up the findings of the study, practical recommendations and areas for future research.

The main difference between a PhD thesis and the theses submitted for undergraduate and master's degrees is that a PhD thesis typically reports on a series of studies that investigate a research problem from different perspectives. At PhD level, candidates would not just describe the methods of their studies but would also discuss methodology, ontological and epistemological issues, and justify the approach taken in their research. The introduction, literature review and methodology chapters are followed by separate chapters for each study and an overall discussion synthesising the findings and a conclusion chapter. The methodology could be a separate chapter or it could be integrated with the literature review. The chapter for each study would typically state the purpose of the study, description the specific methods and report the findings.

Very good research can be submitted for publication in scientific journals or presentation at scientific conferences. The abstract for a conference is similar to the abstract for a dissertation; it is an overall synopsis of what was done, how it was done and what was found. If an abstract is accepted for podium presentation at a conference, sides need to be produced. A conference presentation may be as short as 5 minutes (BASES, 2023) but is typically around 15 to 2 minutes including questions. Slides should not contain paragraphs of text but instead should include key points, images, charts and summary tables.

Poster presentations are also done at conferences. The poster should include key figures, tables and photographs to convey details of the methods, results and theoretical aspects. The poster can be viewed by others at their leisure and discussed with the researcher informally. Some conferences give poster presenters a few minutes to talk about their research and answer one or two questions.

Journal articles would not typically include a full literature review. The introduction is, instead, a focused background to the specific research problem.

The methods and results follow, and the discussion and conclusions may be merged into a single section. There are often word limits to journal articles and often the full set of results presented in a thesis cannot be included. Instead, the key results tables and charts are included to keep the paper concise. Journals have author guidelines that should be consulted by researchers submitting papers to the journal. Some journals publish review articles, including systematic reviews, as well as original research papers.

There are various referencing systems in use such as the Harvard system used in the current textbook. Whatever referencing style is used, it should be used consistently. When referring to published work, we need to refer to it accurately when discussing what was found and the methods used.

Conclusions

This introductory chapter of this book has covered what performance analysis is, and how it is used in coaching, media, judging and academic contexts. This chapter has provided a rationale for the use of performance analysis support services in coaching contexts based on the limitations of coach recall of events. The activities that occur within performance analysis support can still be represented by the early model of Franks and Miller (1986) which has been discussed within this chapter. Sports performance research uses performance analysis data collection methods within descriptive studies. There is a growing number of successful performance analysis research teams and research is becoming more international and applied to a greater range of sports. However, there remain concerns about the quality of some research submitted for journal publication. There is still a great need for research into the effectiveness of applied performance analysis in coaching using in-depth case studies.

2 Sports performance data and information

Introduction

The terms "data" and "information" are not terms that can be used interchangeably. When we have a process, the input to that process is referred to as "data" and the output from that process is referred to as "information". The purpose of the process is to transform data into summary information. We may have pipelines of processes where the output from one process is passed onto the next process. Therefore, the information produced by the first process would be considered as data with respect to the next process in the pipeline. The processes involved in a sports performance analysis system may be manual tasks, automated tasks or a combination of both.

In the first edition of this book, performance analysis was represented as a largely reductive process commencing with the actual sports performance and gradually reducing the wealth of complex data within the performance to a set of quantitative variables that summarised key aspects of the performance (O'Donoghue, 2015: 57). The main reason for such a representation of performance analysis was because of the emphasis of the book on students completing research assessments analysing sports performance. Research in the area of performance analysis typically leads to quantitative results about performances that are presented in thesis, research article, poster or slide form. When performance analysis is used in coaching contexts, the process does not stop when match statistics have been produced. The match statistics tend to dictate which areas of performance need closer attention and which video sequences need to be examined when providing feedback to players. Therefore, Figure 2.1 provides an alternative representation of the use of different types of data and information in sports performance analysis. This will be used to introduce the different types of data and information used in performance analysis before this chapter continues to discuss these in detail.

The top left of Figure 2.1 shows that the actual performance is the starting point of the analysis. Sports performance is complex and involves multiple different types of data. The events recorded on match videos contain vast amounts of data in each video frame, with additional complexity being added as player actions take place over successive video frames. However, these

DOI: 10.4324/9781003375463-2

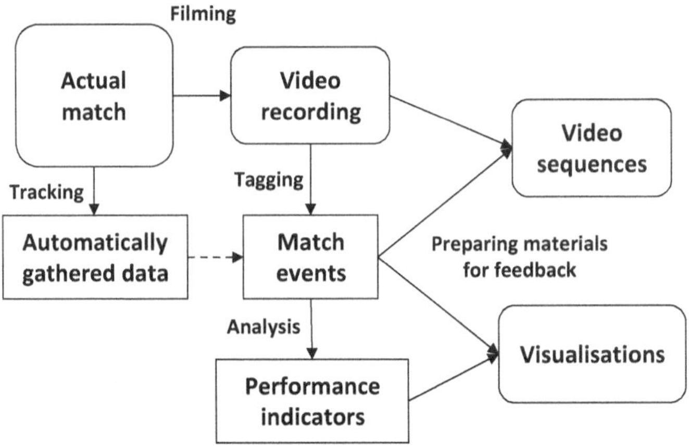

Figure 2.1 Data and information within sports performance analysis.

two-dimensional portrayals of the match, together with sound recorded on the video, miss a great deal of things that happen during the match. Firstly, the match video may not display the entire playing area in a game sport, but instead follow the on-the-ball action. Thus, much off-the-ball movement may not be represented in the match video. Secondly, a lot of what is being experienced by players during matches is not represented on a match video. Consider competing in sport yourself, and consider a particularly challenging performance where difficulties had to be overcome to achieve your goal. Try to remember what it felt like and what you were thinking at the time. These thoughts and feelings are not represented on video recordings, although body language can give some indications (Furley et al., 2015). Figure 2.1 shows automatically gathered data such as player movement trajectories which can be captured using GPS or image-based player tracking technology (Leser and Roemer, 2015). Automatically gathered data can also include heart rate measurements recorded during actual performance. Where both the player and the ball are tracked, it is possible for software to automatically determine some match events like passes and dribbles (Lames, 1994). Match event data is typically created by analysts tagging match videos. This further reduces the data from what has been recorded on the video to a list of match events. Event records typically classify the event type (pass, shot, tackle, etc.) and may also include descriptor fields for the team and player performing the event, the outcome of the event and possibly the area of the field the event was performed in. There may be additional data coded depending on the requirements of the squad. The data within event records are typically categorical, and the event records together form an event list which can be exported for further processing spreadsheet packages. Commercial video analysis packages often provide an analysis feature to reduce the event data into a matrix of events by descriptors. This takes the categorical data in the event list and produces more quantitative information, namely the frequencies of events where different descriptors have been used. Further processing of these data can combine frequency data to produce performance indicators that reflect the whole performance rather than individual events. For example, if the matrix includes the number of passes performed successfully and the number of passes performed unsuccessfully, then two performance indicators can be produced. These are the total number of passes played and the percentage of passes that are played successfully.

At this point, Figure 2.1 differs to the pipeline of data processing activity in the first edition of this book (O'Donoghue, 2015: 57). The performance indicators can alert analysts and coaches to areas of good play and areas requiring attention. Relevant video sequences need to be selected for players to discuss during debriefing sessions. Players and coaches will discuss the areas of play displayed on these video sequences in much greater depth than the way the performance is represented by quantitative information. It would be counterproductive tagging such detail because it would delay feedback being provided and the details are shown on the video sequences anyway. Essentially, what is being depicted in Figure 2.1 is a reductive approach that generates performance indicators that can be used to target the richer in-depth analysis of video sequences that occur during feedback sessions. Figure 2.1 also shows that additional visualisations can be produced to help communicate areas of performance to players.

Qualitative data in sports performance analysis

Qualitative data are typically complex and include visual patterns, video, images, words, feelings, thoughts and emotions. The meanings of such data are interpreted by those analysing them and typically rely on personal judgement. Much of these data are lost as performances are analysed by tagging videos with events.

Qualitative observation

Non-participant observation is used in both coaching and sports performance analysis. Non-participant observation is where the researcher or analyst overtly investigates the behaviour of interest without personally engaging in it. This kind of observational analysis has been used in coaching and predate the use of notational analysis (Hayes, 1997). Coaches typically observe performance during training and competition, evaluating athlete performance drawing on knowledge and experience. The observation is not restricted by the coding templates typically used by match analysts. During training, the coach has the option to intervene and provide feedback periodically. During competition, the scope for intervention and providing feedback may be limited to intervals between match periods and time-outs.

Sports performance analysis has been portrayed as an objective means of providing accurate information to coaches and players. However, there are sports performance analysis tasks where behaviours are classified using subjective judgement during the data entry process. Consider the soccer defender wishing to reach a ball on the wing of the defensive third of the field and play the ball up field. An opposing striker also wishes to reach the ball and play a cross into the penalty area. As the players reach the ball, the ball is played by the defender, striking the opposing striker's leg and goes out for a throw in to the defender's team. Neither player achieved their objective but some systems force the analyst to record such a one-on-one duel as being won by one player or the other (Gerisch and Reicheldt, 1991).

Once video sequences are observed by players, more unrestricted observation and analysis allows the extent to which each player achieved their goal to be considered. Alternative options available to players will not have been tagged, but can be analysed when players and coaches are viewing video sequences. This allows them to consider whether the option chosen was a good choice or not irrespective of how well the event was performed. Qualitative video observation allows decisions to draw upon all of the audio-visual information available.

Qualitative movement diagnosis

The unrestricted qualitative analysis described previously is also relevant to technique intensive sports. Consider a sprinter during a track training session. The coach can observe, taking in as much information as they can, and mentally noting key feedback points. This is an example of "qualitative movement diagnosis" (Knudson, 2013). Qualitative movement diagnosis is made up of four phases (Knudson, 2013: 1):

- Preparation
- Observation
- Evaluation and Diagnosis
- Intervention

Preparation involves developing knowledge necessary to observe, analyse and intervene. The coach or analyst needs a knowledge of the sport, particularly elements of technique associated with success. Knowledge about the sport can come from direct personal experience, professional development courses, education and scientific research. Knowledge of the sport includes the critical features of the sport, the temporal structure of skills and the relationships between the sport and abilities required for different skills. Knowledge of the sport includes models of performance outcome in terms of movements performed during different stages of skills. For example, Hay (1983) used a hierarchical model of the long jump to show how different aspects contributed to the distance achieved. Knowledge of common faults and how to rectify these also help performance monitoring and feedback. It is also important to have knowledge about the performer, because not all athletes are the same and their individual anthropometric characteristics, attentional style, other psychological factors, physical ability and experience may all require them to perform differently to others in the same sport (Knudson, 2013: 86–87).

Observation is best done when being properly prepared to observe. Understanding the nature of the sport can allow an abstract conceptual model to be used as a guide. Data collection forms can be designed cross-tabulating body component with temporal phases of the event (Gangstead and Beveridge, 1984). These allow notes to be recorded in a systematic way. The causes of performance errors may be far removed from the effects of those errors (Knudson, 2013, p. vii) and it may require repeated observation to identify these causes.

Evaluation and diagnosis consider a range of critical features, prioritising them according to their impact on overall performance and whether they can be corrected in the short term or long term. This may involve comparing the observed performance to an ideal performance (Knudson, 2013: 117). Analysing performance using knowledge of common faults may be more productive for improving technique in beginners (Franks, 1997). As athletes approach expert level, the ideal performance becomes more relevant, allowing subtle differences to the athlete's technique to be identified (Franks, 1997).

The intervention stage involves providing augmented feedback (Knudson, 2013: 138).

Packages such as Dartfish (Dartfish, Fribourg, Switzerland) contain features that aid analysis and feedback. Split screen views can be used to view a performance from different angles once videos have been synchronised. Alternatively, the split screen view can be used to display two different performances for the purpose of comparison. These could be two performances by the same athlete or performances of two different athletes. Delayed playback of recorded video can be used in training, competition or physical education settings. An example of delayed video feedback is the "in-the-action" facility of the Dartfish$_{TM}$ system that allows an athlete to perform a skill and then view their performance 30 s later when it is displayed on a computer screen. The Simulcam$_{TM}$ facility of Dartfish allows different performances at the same venue to be shown with one superimposed on the other (Dartfish, n.d.-a). This allows a more direct comparison than a split screen view showing the two performances. The image processing software produces a single image where a blended view is produced by compensating for different camera angles used in the two original video sequences. Stromotion is a feature of the Dartfish package that produces a single image containing a series of static images of an athlete, or object, displayed on a background constructed from background images within the individual frames of the original video sequence (Dartfish, n.d.-b). For a more in-depth coverage of "qualitative movement diagnosis", we recommend Knudson's (2013) book on the subject which has been referred to on several occasions in the current subsection.

Images

As mentioned in the previous subsection, Stromotion can produce a single image containing multiple images of the athlete as they move across the sports arena. Producing such an image requires some highly sophisticated image processing, but the end product is an image that is useful feedback for athletes. Images of sports performance can be analysed without any additional processing. For example, images of the hitting phase in tennis have been used to study the visual gaze of elite tennis players (Lafont, 2008). Lafont (2008) makes a very good point that some key actions in sport are performed in milliseconds and, therefore, cannot be analysed possibly by watching video. A static image that has been photographed with a high-speed camera can avoid blurring and allow important features of movement to be discussed while examining the photograph. Still images can also be saved from videos of team game performance to allow tactical positioning to be analysed. Chapter 7 of this book covers telestration where video frames can be augmented with symbols highlighting key movements, areas and positioning (Jones et al., 2020).

The "inner athlete"

The thoughts and emotions experienced by athletes during sports performance cannot be directly observed from video recordings of performances. Interviewing athletes about their thoughts and emotions during performance is likely to lead to athletes reporting on experiences of performance in general rather than obtaining information about specific performances. However, Poizat et al. (2013) describe the self-confrontation interview to gain access to athletes' experiences during sports performance. The interview is in the form of a video debriefing, meaning that the athlete can interviewer are watching a video of the performance during the interview. The interviewer encourages the athlete to "relive" the performance and discuss their thoughts and emotions at critical points in the performance. When used in a coaching context, this can help the athlete reflect on performance and develop an understanding of how performance may have deteriorated. The self-confrontational interview also allows the interviewer (whether a coach, analyst, or researcher) to compare their initial perceptions of the performance with the perceptions of the athlete. When used in sports performance analysis research, the data can be analysed to contribute to knowledge of these unseen aspects of actual sports performance.

Quantitative data

Performance variables and action variables

The qualities required for a variable to be considered a performance indicator are discussed later in this chapter. The purpose of the current subsection is to distinguish performance variables and action variables. A performance variable may be a performance indicator, or it might not fulfil all of the criteria to be termed a performance indicator. A performance variable characterises an aspect of the performance; by the performance, we mean the match or at least a substantial period of the match like a quarter or a half. Examples of performance variables in soccer could be:

- The number of shots on goal.
- The number of short passes.
- The number of long passes.
- The percentage of short passes that reach a teammate.
- The percentage of long passes that reach a teammate.
- The number of tackles attempted.
- The percentage of tackles that are successful.
- The number of aerial balls attempted.
- The percentage of aerial balls won.
- The percentage of time the team is in possession of the ball.

All of these performance indicators take numerical values. Action variables, on the other hand, are about individual match events. The events could happen in instantaneous moments of the match or take place over some non-zero duration of time. Examples of instantaneous events could be passes if they are tagged at the moment the passer strikes the ball. There is also the possibility that some could legitimately tag passes from the moment the ball is played until the ball is received by a teammate, intercepted or goes out of the field of play. However, this alternative tagging approach might prolong the time it takes to tag the match and delay time to feedback. Examples of events performed over non-zero duration are possessions, especially if we wish to determine a total for possession time from the tagged data. Action variables typically have categorical values, though it is recognised that numerical timings are recorded for event instances. Examples of action variables related to the previous list of performance variables are (with values in parentheses):

- Team (home or away team).
- Event (shot, short pass, long pass, tackle, aerial attempt).
- Outcome (successful, unsuccessful).
- Possession (home team possession, away team possession, stoppage).

The performance variables are expressed in terms of these action variables. For example, the percentage of long passes that reach a teammate simply divides the number of events that are long passes and where the outcome is successful by the number of events that are long passes and expresses this as a percentage. This would typically be done for the home and away team separately. Once these relationships between all performance variables and action variables are set up, we do not need to define the performance variables any further. It is only necessary to define the action variables. However, objectivity is not guaranteed by using operational definitions. Achieving objectivity for the action variables, and hence for the performance variables as well, requires training for system users.

Automated data collection

Quantitative data are measured rather than judged. The first type of quantitative data we will discuss are data that are gathered using automated systems. Hawk-eye (Hawk-eye Innovations, Basingstoke, UK) have developed systems for ball tracking in sport that are used in tennis and cricket. The system has been used for both officiating and media purposes. Ball tracking uses images from multiple cameras within triangulation algorithms. At each point in time, two-dimensional frames from different cameras are used to form a three-dimensional space, calculating the ball's location within this. Analysing these video frames over time allows the flight of the ball to be calculated. The first edition of this book explained how a tennis ball might not make contact with the ground in any of the video frames analysed, even when the frame rate is 500 Hz (O'Donoghue, 2015: 38–39). Therefore, the location at which the ball contacts the ground must be calculated using predictive models of ball flight given the frames that have been recorded. Hawk-eye's website has reported the average error for the location of where the ball bounces to be 3.6 mm (Hawk-eye, n.d.). There are other examples of ball tracking used during media coverage with additional products for player use. One example is the Flightscope system (Flightscope, Orlando, FL) used in golf where ball trajectories are tracked using Doppler radar (Flightscope, n.d.).

Hawk-eye have also developed the goal-line technology used in soccer and Gaelic football. Goal-line technology also requires predictive algorithms to estimate whether the whole of the ball has crossed the whole of the goal line in a game of soccer. This is because it is possible that the whole of the ball could cross the whole of the goal line without this being recorded in a single frame (O'Donoghue, 2015: 40). Despite the data collected by these systems being highly quantitative, they can be presented in as a pattern allowing more subjective analysis by users. For example, Figure 2.2 represents the type of image that can be output from Hawk-eye for use in officiating or by the media. Other visualisations in cricket include "wagon wheel" diagrams that show where balls are played and ball flight images for bowling.

Technology, such as global positioning systems (GPS) systems, has also been developed to track player movement. The Catapult system (Catapult Sports, Melbourne, Victoria, Australia) integrates GPS data with heart rate data and accelerometer data within a reasonably unobtrusive device that can be worn by players, located near the subscapular. The data can be transferred wirelessly to laptop computers, iPads or iPhones on the sideline of the playing

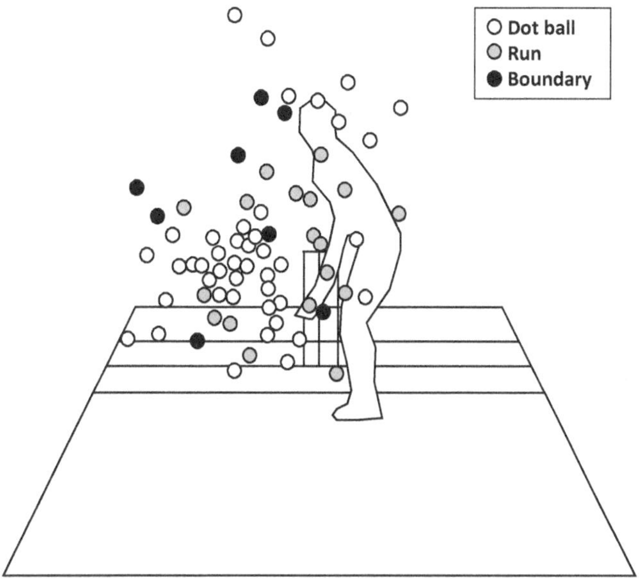

Figure 2.2 Representation of balls faced by a cricket batsman.

area in real time. The Vector S7 device operates at 400 Hz and the data can be integrated with ball tracking data. The system can also operate indoors due to its LPS (Local positioning system) capability.

The main advantage of totally automated systems is that there is no subjective human classification of movement or behaviour during the process of data gathering. This does not necessarily mean that systems are accurate, but it does mean that they are free of perceptual errors that can be made by human operators. Automated object and player tracking systems offer accurate recording of larger volumes of information than would be the case with human operators. There are also some limitations in using automatic object and player tracking systems. Object tracking systems, such as Hawk-eye, need to be set up carefully as any slight misplacement of a camera can lead to inaccurate recording of ball location. Where an automatic player tracking system records player location accurately and frequently (for example, at 25 Hz), the actual path travelled by the player is unknown meaning the tracking system must estimate the path between sampled locations based on assumptions. Many player tracking systems record player location without recording whether the player is moving forwards, shuffling backwards and skipping sideways. Where player tracking systems don't distinguish between forward, backward and sideways movement, the amount of time spent performing high speed running (5.5 $m.s^{-1}$ or faster) will under-estimate the amount of high intensity activity being performed. Other high intensity activity that would not be recognised includes vertical movement to compete for aerial balls.

Quantitative analysis of qualitative data

In the first edition of this book, there was a section on "traditional notational analysis". Notational analysis was a term initially used in the 20th century for manual methods of recording sports performance data such as tally systems. The advent of computerised systems integrating video with match event data led to a distinction being made between manual and computerised notational analysis. The term notation suggests a manual use of shorthand symbols to record data. Since the turn of the century, the term "performance analysis" has become more commonly used than "notational analysis". Indeed, eight years after the first edition of this book was published, we can consider the use of commercial video tagging packages to be traditional match analysis, with more contemporary systems using more advanced technology. Match analysis involves subjective judgement at the point of data collection. Consider a soccer match where a player contacts with the ball and the ball is then picked up by a teammate. The analyst does not believe a pass to the given receiver was intended and that this was just a touch of the ball. However, the analyst is also wondering whether this should be counted as a pass because the ball was successfully transferred between two players on the same team. Whatever is entered will be recorded as a categorical event type (pass or touch) within the match event list. The data will be analysed producing quantitative information about the number of touches and the number of passes. However, at the point of data collection when the analyst tagged the event, there is a subjective decision being made as to whether the event was a touch or a pass. The process involves analyst perception of behaviour. There are ways to improve the objectivity of traditional match analysis systems through guidance to observers. For example, we might be clear that any ball transfer from a player to a teammate should be recorded as a pass. There are some definitions which are quite specific but which cannot be implemented with precision by a human observer. For example, we might specify that a long pass should involve the ball travelling at least 10 m. The issue here is that while such a definition can be agreed, it is difficult to tell, when observing the match, if a pass of about 10 m is just under or just over 10 m.

The main advantage of traditional match analysis is that it manages the complexity of sports performance, creating an abstract representation of the performance that aids analysis and feedback. Traditional match analysis combines quantitative techniques while also benefitting from expert observer judgement and experience. There are also disadvantages to using traditional match analysis. The level of reliability is typically lower than when automated data collection is used. For example, the time at which a rally in tennis ends may be delayed by the analyst identifying this during observation and clicking on the appropriate button of the code template. There are also times where precise definitions can result in measuring something other than what we intended. Consider a system to record rallies in tennis. We could objectively define the rally as being over when it has ended according to the rules of tennis. The rally may end where an error is played (the ball strikes the net or lands somewhere other than the opponent's half of the court) or a winner is played (the ball lands in the opponent's half of the court and bounces for a second time before the opponent can retrieve it). If a player hits the ball high in the air so it is obviously not going to land in, then the rally is effectively over and both players will be able to relax and prepare for the next point. However, the rally is not recorded as having ended until the shot actually lands out. Therefore, the overall time spent in rallies will be an over-estimate of the high intensity work done by the players.

Self-report variables

Earlier in this chapter, we discussed how self-confrontational interviews allow athletes thoughts and emotions during sports performance to be explored. There are also more quantitative self-report variables that can be derived from actual sports performance. For example, a study used swimmers' and table tennis players' self-reported competitive anxiety, confidence and momentum perceptions while they were observing videos of recent performances (Briki et al., 2012). The participants viewed the video on separate occasions to report momentum and the psychological variables. They identified the start and ends of periods of perceived positive momentum. They then used a mouse to dynamically enter levels of the psychological variables from "not at all" to "very much so" while watching the video of their performance. Cognitive anxiety, somatic anxiety and self-confidence were then plotted against time within the table tennis or swimming performance. A separate chart plotted the relationships between these different variables over time within the performance; hence there were three lines, one for each pair of variables being correlated. They found the relationships between these variables to be more consistent in table tennis than in swimming. There are other psychological variables, such as the mood (McNair et al., 1971) that could be tracked in a similar way during post-match video observation. The key distinction to the work of Poizat and colleagues (2013) is that these variables are quantitative and can be analysed statistically.

Performance indicators

Figure 2.1 shows that in team games performance indicators are ultimately derived from action variables that have been created during video tagging. This does not necessarily mean that any summary variable derived from event data is a performance indicator. Variables must possess important qualities to be termed performance indicators. These qualities are validity, having an objective measurement procedure, a known scale of measurement, and a means of interpretation. The following subsections discuss these qualities in turn.

Validity

A variable is valid if it represents an important and relevant aspect of the performance and if the variable itself is a valid measure of the aspect. Ultimately, this means the variable must be useful and there are decisions about preparation and tactics that can be made using the variable. There are five different types of validity that are relevant in sports performance analysis (O'Donoghue, 2010: 150–155). These are summarised below:

- Logical validity (or face validity) is where the variable is obviously valid, for example, the 10,000 m time of a 10,000 m runner.
- Content validity is relevant to performance profiles which are discussed in greater detail in Chapter 10 of this book. A performance profile has content validity if it consists of performance indicators that cover all relevant aspects of performance.
- Criterion validity is where a performance variable is related to some gold standard measure such as the result of the match. Therefore, the performance variable is either associated with the winning margin, time or distance achieved or is a variable where winning and losing performers have clearly different values.
- Construct validity applies where some measure is not directly observable within a performance but is created; for example, the Eagle rating (Bracewell et al., 2003). Such a construct has construct validity if it clearly distinguishes between performers of known different ability levels.
- Decision accuracy is where the variable can at least distinguish between winners and losers of matches even though the actual recorded value might not be considered a valid measure of performances of different qualities.

Not all performance indicators are related to the outcome of the match. Some may represent the style of play rather than the effectiveness of play. Tactical indicators, for example, represent the style of play irrespective of the success with which the style of play is performed. Soccer teams using a high press, when the opposition has the ball, may exist in the top and bottom of a league. Similarly, teams who adopt alternative defensive tactics may also exist at the top and bottom of a soccer league. Consider a situation where we have a valid and reliable way of counting when a team is pressing. A performance indicator could be the number of opposition possessions where the team is pressing. There may be no difference for this performance indicator between the average team in the top half of the league and the average team in the bottom half of the league. This reflects that the proportion of teams adopting this tactic and the extent to which they adopt it may be similar between the teams in the two halves of the league. This does not mean that it is invalid because the purpose of this indicator is not to distinguish successful and unsuccessful teams but to distinguish teams adopting different defensive styles. The style adopted by an opposing team is important to understand when preparing to play against them. Hence, tactical indicators can be performance indicators.

Objective measurement process

The previous subsection on validity used an example of pressing in soccer. There was a big "if" with this example which was whether we could reliably identify where a team was pressing. A variable is objective if its value is independent of a given observer's opinion. Some automatically measured variables are objective because they do not involve any human judgement during data collection. Such variables include ball and player tracking variables, heart rate response and some biomechanical variables. The objectivity achieved at the data recording level means that any performance indicator derived from such data can also be assumed to be objective. For example, if player locations are objectively measured every 25th of a second then any speed distribution variables, or distance variables derived from these measurements will also be objective.

Where data are collected by analysts tagging match videos, some variables may be made objective by devolving decisions to the match officials. Therefore, even if the analyst believes an official's decision is incorrect, they record the official's decision anyway because this is what has happened in the match. This means that the observers will not be exercising any subjective judgement over rule infringements or whether scores have occurred.

There are other action variables that need to be classified by analysts while they are tagging matches. Some behaviours may be more matter-of-fact than others. For example, an analyst is usually able to see where a player has passed the ball off the field of play. There may be some other occasions, where it is not obvious whether the ball was last touched by a player or an opposing player before going out of play. However, in such a situation, the analyst can enter the decision made by the match officials. Returning to the example where a player obviously plays the ball out, the analyst may be required to classify this error as a forced or an unforced error. This can be difficult because it requires the analyst to make judgements about the degree of difficulty of the situation and the pressure being applied by opposing players. Analyst judgements may not only be required to assess the competence with which skills are performed but they may also need to classify different techniques. For example, the flat, slice and kick serve techniques in tennis may be difficult for analysts to distinguish unless they have a good knowledge of tennis. This example raises an interesting point about the use of operational definitions. A tennis expert could write down some definitions for flat, slice and kick serves and guidelines for distinguishing these. However, the definitions may be in use terminology that needs to be further defined leading to a large volume of text. It is still possible that an observer, who is not familiar with tennis, would not be able to fully understand these definitions. It is also possible that an observer, who is familiar with tennis, would not use the definitions as they already consider themselves able to distinguish these three serving styles. The same problem occurs in field games where we may wish to distinguish between player-to-player marking and zonal defence. Is it worth even trying to define at what point a defensive pattern becomes zonal (or player-to-player marking) with respect to the location of the opposing players? If distances or areas are mentioned in such definitions, would we actually be able to accurately measure these when observing match videos? Are experts who are knowledgeable in the sport able to recognise different defence styles being applied from visual information in the absence of operational definitions? Would they be able to describe the processes they use to recognise such defensive patterns?

Given that the use of operational definitions may be counterproductive for some action variables, the role of subjective behaviour classification in sports performance analysis should be recognised. Where subjective human classification is involved in the data collection process, it is necessary to demonstrate the level of objectivity of the data collection process using inter-operator agreement studies. This would be where two trained observers analyse a performance, or possibly several performances, and the level of agreement between the data they collect is assessed. The kappa statistic can be used to cross-tabulate the two sets of events and determine the level of agreement adjusting for the expected level of agreement by chance (O'Donoghue, 2015: 191–193). Note, where two observers have differing numbers of events, it is necessary to time match these and insert null events where one observer has recorded and event but the other has not (O'Donoghue and Holmes, 2015: 225–228). This type of reliability analysis is about the data at the event level. It may be more important to assess if the resulting variables indicators are reliable. Evaluating the reliability of numerical performance variables would require multiple matches to be analysed to ensure that both systematic bias and random error components of error are represented. Systematic bias is where one observer has a greater tendency to count behaviour as a particular event than another observer. If these two observers were to look at multiple matches, this difference would not be uniform, but the average difference could be calculated. This average difference is the systematic bias. Differences between corresponding observations that are greater than or lower than the systematic bias include random error. This means that it is possible for exact agreement for one particular match due to the systematic bias being cancelled out by random error. If a single match is analysed, this might happen and the observers would not realise it because the systematic bias would not have been calculated from a single match. Therefore, multiple match reliability studies avoid situations where a single match reliability study yields 100% agreement because some errors in the collection of some events are cancelled out by opposite errors when collecting other events. Reliability is important at both the event level and the performance indicator level. The performance indicators may influence the overall assessment of the performance and dictate the video sequences to be used in feedback.

However, players will still be concerned if individual events they perform are not analysed reliably.

Known scale of measurement

Performance indicators need to have known scales of measurement. Knowing the full range of values that a performance indicator can take assists in its interpretation. It is not always possible to set an upper limit for the values of frequency variables in the way that can be done for percentage conversion rates. A further issue with frequency variables is that some sports have varying match lengths, especially when matches are structured into sets like in tennis and volleyball. In these sports, it might be better to express frequency per set rather than the overall frequency for a variable. Of course, some sets may be longer than others as well which might warrant further adjustments so that frequency data are scaled with respect to match length. Turning to success measures, consider the percentage of passes that a soccer player successfully plays to a teammate. We might reasonably expect this to range between 50% and 90% with the possibility of some performances being outside this range. A further issue is that defenders and midfielders tend to play more successful passes than forwards (Redwood-Brown et al., 2019). Therefore, the range of values may differ for players of different positions. The meaningful range of values for some performance indicators can be narrow. For example, the percentage of lineouts where possession is retained is 87% and 85% for the top four teams and bottom four teams respectively in English Premier League rugby (Migdalski and Stone, 2019).

Means of interpretation

When we discussed the scale of measurement for a performance indicator, we suggested that the range of values we might expect to see for the percentage of passes in soccer, that are successfully played to a teammate, varies depending on the positional role of the player. When interpreting a performance indicator's value, we not only need to know what are high and low values but we also need to know what are good values. It is preferable to achieve high values for outcome indicators such as the number of points won in a set of tennis. There are other indicators such as the number of unforced errors made where lower values are preferable. Then, there are performance indicators where optimal values are better. For example, the percentage of passes reaching a teammate in a game of soccer could be too high to be good, if the success rate is being achieved by playing safe passes and failing to attempt more risky penetrative passes that could lead to scoring opportunities. Figure 2.3 is a representation of this concept. This is a speculative model that requires more research to explore. When examining passing data in soccer, it is difficult to obtain a pattern such as the one portrayed in Figure 2.3. There are a number of reasons for this. Firstly, when an individual pass is played, it

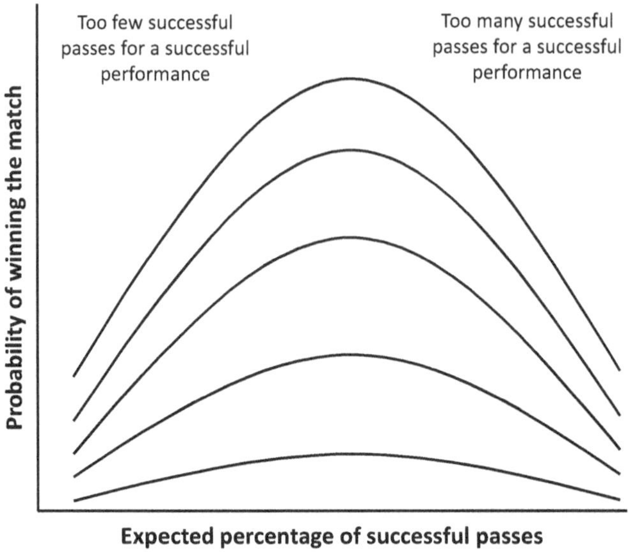

Figure 2.3 Conceptual model of passing and success in soccer.

will either be successful or not. At the action variable level, it is categorical. We do not see the level of risk or the probability of success for the pass. All of these individual passes can be combined to provide a numerical performance indicator for the percentage of passes that were played successfully. Where there are enough passes, this percentage may reflect the level of risk taken when playing passes. However, the probability of success of passing attempts has not actually been gauged when the data were collected. Any analysis to try and retrospectively study this concept would need to control for the quality of teams within matches.

A further issue in interpreting performance indicators is that some performance indicators may be related to each other. For example, one might consider the number of double faults played in tennis to be a performance indicator where lower values are better. However, a tennis player avoiding double faults by playing safer second serves may also reduce the number of points they win when they have to take a second serve. This is because a safer second serve is easier for the receiving player to return and thus would set the whole point up differently than if a second serve was played with greater speed and closer to the edge of the service box. Therefore, when interpreting a performance indicator such as the number of double faults, it may be necessary to ask if the number of double faults played is tolerable given the number of second serve points won when the second serve is in, especially the number of second serve points won where the server did not have to play a second shot.

Norms can also be used in the interpretation of performance indicator values. Norms have been used in the interpretation of anthropometric variables such as body mass index (CDC, 2022). These norms allow people to compare someone's body mass index to the relevant population of people based on age and gender. This works for reasonably stable variables such as anthropometric variables. The issue with sports performance variables is that they can fluctuate on a week to week basis with the largest factor influencing performance being the quality of opposition. Therefore, norms for performance indicators in sport need to be established for different types of matches based on the quality of the teams involved (O'Donoghue et al., 2008).

Conclusions

This chapter has distinguished between the terms "data" and "information" and discussed the various forms of data used in sports performance analysis. Ultimately, sports performances contain very rich complex data that need to be reduced to a form allowing efficient analysis. The current chapter has described how the actual performance is firstly reduced to a video representation, then a list of events containing quantitative data, before finally being summarised as performance indicators representing the performance. These quantitative data serve to direct the attention of coaches and players to particular elements of the game. This re-introduces video level data that expert coaches and players can discuss without the restrictions of quantitative variables. The final part of this chapter covers performance indicators, and the qualities required for a performance variable to be classed as a performance indicator.

3 What to analyse?

Introduction

Irrespective of an analyst's ability to operate video analysis software, performance analysis will be meaningless unless the relevant information is produced. This chapter discusses the various types and qualities of information, and how they can be selected to evaluate a sporting performance. After all, the aim of performance analysis is to provide objective information on performances in training and in competition (O'Donoghue, 2015); to do that, we must first have a clear understanding of what information is relevant to both the athlete and coach and secondly how it can be collected.

The What It Takes To Win (WITTW) approach will also be discussed later in this chapter. An overview of how performance analysts integrate into multidisciplinary teams, working to support athletes alongside other sport science specialists. Taking the UK Sports Institute (UKSI) as an example, expert practitioners will work closely together, thus enabling a support strategy for athletes to compete at the highest level (UK Sports Institute, 2023).

Sport performance and approaches

The purpose of sport performance analysis is to gather unbiased information on an individual or team performance. Through the creation of an analysis system, objective data (statistics) and video feedback can be produced for performances to inform the coaching process. Its distinct difference from other sport science disciplines is that actual performance is analysed (O'Donoghue, 2015), whether that be in a training or match environment. The combination of objective data and video clips is a powerful feedback tool; the data accurately informing participants of what has happened and the associated video sequences providing the context of the situation with further details of how the event actually occurred. As an example, consider the investigation of passing sequences for midfield players in soccer. It was reported that Player A had a 100% (33 out of 33 passes) pass completion rate, with Player B reporting a 91% (21 out of 23 passes) result. In isolation and solely relying on data, it is evident that Player A had a more successful

DOI: 10.4324/9781003375463-3

performance and had a greater involvement with receiving and transferring the ball within the game. Further exploration into the data and supported by video, it was identified that 33% (11 passes) of Player A's passes were short lateral passes played deep within their own half. In comparison, the associated video clips highlighted that 30% (7 passes) of Player B's passes were forward and more direct passes played higher up the pitch. This allowed the team to get behind the defence and into more attacking areas. In summary, objective data combined with video feedback provides a holistic overview of performance. This can be used to review own, preview opposition and develop strategies for future performances. In support of analysing performance and obtaining an account of events, Laird and Waters (2008) reported that qualified and experienced coaches only recalled 59.2% of events accurately from 45 minutes of a soccer match; this reinforces the need for analysts to objectively measure performance and provide accurate feedback to coaching teams. The need for sport performance analysis is clear, it will provide an accurate account of events undertaken in both training and performance environments. The combination of objective data and video sequences will support the development of athletes and the decisions of coaches. Without an accurate record of performance, whether that be a sole resource of data or video or a combination of both, it is likely that interpretations of performance will be misinformed and based solely on subjective recollections of events. Consider the impact of making a substitution based on performance metrics, for example, tackles made and missed or metres gained? Now consider the consequence of making decisions without this information. What is the impact of this decision? A change was needed but was the correct athlete substituted from what you recall has happened in the game? Was anything missed? Aside from coaching decisions, the feedback process also becomes vague without an accurate record of events, particularly as time passes between actual performance and review sessions. Using the substituted athlete as an example, valuable factual information can be shared on the decision if the performance was analysed. Whole team meetings can also be more meaningful when performances have been reviewed. In place of using the memory of individuals to explain situations and events that occurred, analysed video clips and objective data can be shared. This firstly promotes discussions on what has happened and why? Secondly, this provides a platform to develop strategies to overcome similar events, should they occur in future performances.

When implementing analysis, it is firstly important to consider environments. Analysis can take place live in-match, post-match or within training environments, with a focus on our own and/or opposition performances. Naturally, a strength of conducting analysis during a match which is shared continually with coaches, is that it provides an opportunity to make immediate changes. This is in contrast to post-match analysis whereby a fixture has ended, and the focus for coaches and athletes diverts to reflecting on the performance, preparing for training sessions and upcoming fixtures.

A strength of post-match analysis in comparison to live analysis, however, is the opportunity to add greater detail to events. With time being more generous, footage of performances can be rewound and replayed allowing for additional variables to be added to objective data already collected. Whilst analysis during and post-performances leaves no opportunity for interruption with competitors, analysis during training sessions is deemed more flexible. Within these environments, performances can be interrupted by coaches with interventions to review objective data and video footage of drills. This provides an opportunity for athletes to evaluate their executions before repeating. Regardless of environment, the development of an analysis system is a skill in itself and the data collection process must be well-defined to ensure accurate results are presented to coaches and athletes. In this procedure, it is important that the performance analyst remains impartial and holds no preconceived opinion when collecting evidence, parking the subjectiveness of events and gathering objective information which can presented to coaches and athletes for review.

It has been established above that objective data and video sequences can be gathered in a range of environments. So, it is now important that we divert our attention to 'What we might analyse?'. When quantifying performances, which is the investigation of actual sports performances or performance in training (O'Donoghue, 2009), we must firstly consider the approaches. Hughes (1998) acknowledged five purposes to quantify performance, and these are listed in Table 3.1.

Prior to discussing these in greater detail, it must be noted that approaches are suitable in both individual and team sports as well as individual performances within team sports.

Tactical analysis is typically related to analysing the wider strategies used by players and teams. This involves the evaluation of events to determine if any patterns are detectable based on players involved, location of events, set-up of certain plays or time in match. Using rugby as an example, lineout set-up and calls are usually decided based on the variables listed above, i.e., depending on the current match score, location of lineout and lineout success in the game so far, a certain type of lineout call may be made. This would

Table 3.1 Five approaches to quantify performance with examples (Hughes, 1998)

Approach	*Examples*
Tactical Analysis	Final third entries types, individual contributions, team strategy.
Analysis of Technique	Swimming stroke, tennis serves, hooker throw.
Analysis of Effectiveness	Effectiveness of skill, pass competition rates, effectiveness of tactics.
Analysis of Decision Making	Player decisions in games, coaching decisions, referee decisions.
Movement Analysis	Movement of the ball, dance/gymnastic routines, GPS tracking.

then determine the length of ball thrown (front, middle or back pod) and the number of players involved in the lineout. Once this step has been executed successfully and the ball has been received by the intended recipient, further tactical analysis can be carried out on subsequent phases. Tactical analysis can be carried out on our own performances or it can be used to evaluate opposition performances. Using the rugby example above, counter strategies can be developed in an attempt to overcome opposing teams, should these patterns be identified prior to or during the match. The key here though is not to be too obvious and let the opposition know that you have cracked their code!

Analysis of technique considers the method of the skill and the way it has been executed. This is to ensure the athlete is as efficient and as successful as possible in performing the skill, balanced with negating the chance of injury. Changes to technique may be introduced should an execution need refining or during rehabilitation from injury. This approach has naturally been attributed to individual sports and skills, such as the tennis serve, long jump, deadlift or a swimming stroke, yet it must be noted that technique analysis is also important in team sports. Whilst team sports align themselves to tactical analysis, skills such as the hooker throw in rugby union, drag flick in field hockey and shooting in netball are examples of skills that require technical support to ensure they are executed well.

Technical effectiveness considers the skill but also how well they have been performed. Linking into technique analysis, certain skills can be measured in terms of success, i.e., the success of the first serve in tennis or the accuracy of the hooker throw in rugby union. Contrary to technique analysis, technical effectiveness does not take into consideration the technical movement itself. As with most approaches, key performance indicators (KPIs) produced by performance analysts are usually following negotiations with the coaching team. A tennis coach may require detail on the effectiveness of the first serve in relation to the advantage and deuce court, or at times more specifically dividing these zones into wide, body and T (Figure 3.1). This

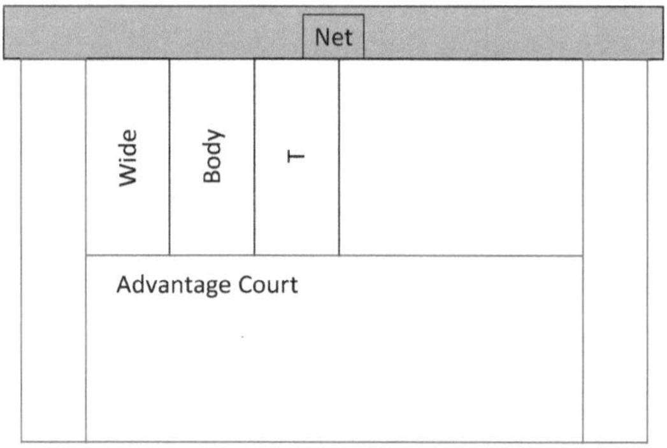

Figure 3.1 Illustration of how technical effectiveness of the tennis serve can be measured in terms of success into the advantage court (wide, body and T zones).

level of detail provides a greater insight into the success of the intended skill, which is to essentially target a specific area of the serving box. This can be measured through KPIs such as:

- % of First Serve Advantage Court, Wide In?
- % of First Serve Advantage Court, Body In?
- % of First Serve Advantage Court, T In?
- % of Second Serve Advantage Court, Wide In?
- % of Second Serve Advantage Court, Body In?
- % of Second Serve Advantage Court, T In?

Depending on participant skill level, the intended skill might be difficult to distinguish. Consider an intermediate tennis player serving to the advantage court with the serve landing on the line between the Body and T zones. Where was the intended location of this serve? Body or T? Of course, a tennis serve is a combination of multiple movements and would naturally benefit from technique analysis support. With a minor skill such as a pass in soccer, the intended action would be more easily identifiable, somewhat regardless of skill level. Environment can also play a part in evaluating the effectiveness of a skill. As discussed above, training environments are more flexible with the freedom to interrupt performances and for skills to be repeatedly played regardless of outcome. Returning to the tennis scenario and within a training environment, the coach may initiate a serving practice to target a specific area of the serving box (e.g., T zone). In this instance, the analysis of the intended skill would become easy to analyse as the intended location is known. This would not be the case in a competition environment though, with no tactical communication permitted between performer and coaching teams. It would therefore be difficult to ascertain the intended location of the skill for a lesser experienced performer. In summary, considerations should be made for the participant's level of experience and also the complexity of the skill performed. Environment types do provide some opportunity to evaluate technical effectiveness with flexibility albeit outside of the constraints of competition and without opposition.

Advancing with experienced tennis players competing in a competition environment, additional key performance indicators related to the technical effectiveness of the serve could include:

- % of First Serve Advantage Court, Wide In and point won
- % of First Serve Advantage Court, Body In and point won
- % of First Serve Advantage Court, T In and point won

This provides an opportunity to evaluate not only the effectiveness of the first serve to the advantage court but also the outcome of the rally. In some scenarios the serve may be an ace, meaning the serve and rally is won instantly by the server. In other scenarios, the serve was in but the rally continues for a series of shots before the opposing player wins the point. In this example, the effectiveness of the serve targeting a particular area is recorded as positive (i.e., % of First Serve Advantage Court, Wide In), yet the overall action variable measuring serve location and point outcome would be recorded as a negative (i.e., % of First Serve Advantage Court, Wide In and Point Won).

Analysis of Decision Making includes the evaluation of tactical choices made by athletes. Whilst the role of the performance analyst in approaches above has been to measure the outcome of an event or skill, this approach evaluates whether the correct decision was made by the athlete at that time. Lorains et al. (2013) described decision making as a key characteristic of expert performance and developed a procedure to evaluate the concept. It would be ill-advised to measure a decision based solely on the outcome; whilst it's agreed the outcome may be successful and ground may be gained in invasion sports such as soccer and rugby union, it is also important to consider other factors. Would another action have been more appropriate or more advantageous to the outcome? Lorains et al. (2013) consider this, developing an approach focusing on match context (score line, player position and player motion), decision making (accuracy of action, options available, defensive pressure on action and disposal time) and skill execution (type of action, effectiveness and error direction).

Movement Analysis incorporates a number of approaches listed above and therefore, why it is discussed last. Movement analysis factors into both tactical and technique analysis, the primarily focused on athlete movement on and off the ball, measuring connections between players in attack or defensive structures. It can also be connected with measuring the physical demands of a sport or event. Time-motion analysis is an approach to measure athlete work rate during performances. Whilst methods vary between Reilly and Thomas (1976), Bloomfield et al. (2004) and O'Donoghue et al. (2005), they do typically share a consensus to categorise movements in an attempt to measure work rate. O'Donoghue et al. (2005) focused on categorising movements into two classifications, Reilly and Thomas (1976) used 7–12 classes, whilst Bloomfield et al. (2004) incorporated directional detail to measure actions completed. Movement analysis on technique focused actions directs its attention to joint and body movements in completing certain skills, whether that be joint angles or acceleration of movements in events such as javelin or hammer throw. In support, Lees (2002) summarised that the earliest approach to evaluating technique was through the principles of movement.

Now with the enhancement of technology, a greater repertoire of methods is available to assist in monitoring athlete movement, these include GPS and LPS monitors as well as wearable devices including smart watches. Specifically, solutions such as Catapult (Catapult, Leeds, UK) have developed sport monitoring units to provide specific insights in a bid to optimise performance, mitigate injury risk and support athletes when returning to play (Catapult, 2023). Their rugby specific solution as an example gathers general metric data such as maximum speed, acceleration, deceleration and player load, along with rugby specific data which includes contact involvements, count of scrums and back in game time. Catapult Vector Clearsky (Catapult, Leeds, UK) also provides a solution to measure performance in the most challenging of environments, whether that be indoor or outdoor performances (Catapult, 2023). The Catapult basketball movement profile gathers data using an algorithm to categorise movement into one of five categories (active, running, dynamic, jumping and settled). This advances on the manual time-motion analysis approaches used by Reilly and Thomas (1976), Bloomfield et al. (2004) and O'Donoghue et al. (2005), driving data collection methods to become automated procedures.

Quality over quantity

The purpose of gathering objective data is to accurately inform athletes and coaches about their performance. KPIs (objective data) can be used to praise actions which have met or exceeded targets, and it allows elements below par to be identified and investigated quickly. KPIs linked with video sequences is a powerful tool, supporting athlete learning and the coaching process. The objectiveness of the data informing 'What has happened' is complemented by the video providing context on 'How and Why' events have taken place. A role of the analyst in this perspective, however, is to manage data collection and expectations of those involved. Quality over quantity of information must remain as an analyst's priority, with consideration of what information can be collected in each environment (in-game, post-game or in training). A contributing factor in generating quality data is understanding the relevance and importance of information and its usefulness in the coaching process. These are traits that aspiring analysts can develop through understanding the sport, the philosophy of the coach and the general analysis environment. These are skills that can be developed by building relationships and using soft skills to communicate with relevant individuals. A technically sound performance analyst will have the ability to gather quality data which encompasses a range of performance variables, yet the recipients of the information may deem it inadequate to the environment. Contrastingly, a well-connected analyst will have the ability to communicate with partners to establish what quality information is needed to inform training and prepare for performance. In the development of a performance analyst, non-technical soft skills associated with the role are often overlooked. Key attributes including how analysts interact with colleagues, the ability to communicate and listen, the ability to manage time to meet deadlines, and the ability to problem solve alone or as a team to identify a practical solution, are all important characteristics to hold. A well-rounded performance analyst will combine their soft skills and hard analyst skills to become a well-connected and competent performance analyst. It is therefore, important when engaging in performance analysis activities, modules or workshops that the development of soft skills is also considered as a learning objective and focus does not solely concentrate on technical skills.

Quality of information refers to the performance variables which are included to fully contextualise an action or event. It is here that on some occasions, further analysis must be conducted on live-analysis databases post-event, when time is more forgiving. In sporting contexts, a first serve to the advantage court and outcome of the rally can be collected during live analysis, yet the exact serve location of T, Body, Wide within the advantage court may need to be added in post-event when footage can be rewound and the result can be accurately recorded. It is the inclusion of this level of information which will emphasise the strengths and limitations of serving strategies. It is important to note that quantity should not be confused with the analysis of multiple matches to develop a profile. When referring to quantity in comparison to quality, it is concerned with simplicity and the generation of masses of generic KPIs. This indicates that a large number of variables have been recorded yet with limited detail or no interaction to the sequence of play. Using soccer as an example, an analyst may find that 800 to 900 passes are performed in a match. This is high in terms of quantity, yet limited in terms of detail. Quality would consider direction of pass, player, success of pass, location pass received, location pass sent or defensive pressure. This level of information can be used to better inform the coaching process.

Standard and detail

When objectively analysing performances, standard of information is important. Firstly, from a judgement perspective using KPIs to draw comparisons between performances; this sets the standard for performances to be measured against. For example, we could be using KPIs to evaluate how Team A compared against Team B this week or how Team A compared against themselves in two consecutive matches. Traditionally, coaching teams and athletes would generate benchmark targets prior to commencing a season, these allowing for performances to be compared. The targets highlight areas of strength and areas below par that require attention. Depending on the method of analysis (manual notation or computerised analysis), statistics can then be reviewed together with video sequences, thus providing further context to objective data. As mentioned previously, the match statistics provide information on 'what' happened, whilst video sequences accompanied by a coach's understanding of tactical strategy, can explain the 'how' and 'why' it occurred.

Standards should also be considered from a reliability stance. Strict protocols must be followed to ensure the standard of information is accurate and reflects coaching terminology and in play events. Operational definitions of performance variables and indicators must be agreed by coaching teams and performance analysts. At times, these may be written descriptions or a repertoire of video clips presenting a clear example of the action and minimising a possibility of misinterpretation.

Coinciding with quality, detail is imperative to support coaching decisions and enhance athlete performances, an aim to provide information to gain an advantage over the opposition. Match statistics are becoming more accessible via broadcast channels and analysis websites, and these are freely available to access during and post-matches. Yet, this information depending on source, can at times be deemed generic, with the accuracy of data collection and operational definitions unknown. Table 3.2 presents a comparison of generic and detailed KPIs across a range of sports.

As presented in Table 3.2, detailed KPIs are crucial to informing the coaching process, as they provide a more focused overview of performance over the production of generic results. Take the indicator of 'number of centre passes' in netball, as an example. Alone, this indicator fails to inform the coaching team of the accuracy or success of the centre passes themselves. Related to count and quantity alone, its only impact is its capability to raise assumptions around centre pass durations. Within a quarter should both teams each take 10 centre passes, the assumption is that each centre pass sequence was prolonged with teams taking time to enter the shooting circle and score a goal; alternatively, a second assumption is that possession changed hands on multiple occasions which equally led to lengthy centre pass sequences. Regardless of either hypothesis, a consequence is that a low number of centre passes were taken within the 15-minute period. On the contrary, should both teams take 18 centre passes in a quarter, it is assumed that play was direct to goal. This is done either by two teams equally contesting and quickly scoring their own centre passes, or one team dominating performance by scoring their own centre pass and turning the opposing centre pass and successfully scoring.

Table 3.2 Examples of generic and detailed KPIs

Sport	*Generic Key Performance Indicator*	*Detailed Key Performance Indicator*
Soccer	% Shots on Target	% Shots on target inside penalty box
	% Final Third Entries	% Final third entries resulting in shot
	% Passes Completed	% Passes completed breaking the line of defence
Tennis	% 1st Serve In	% 1st Serve in when serving to T, Body, Wide
	% Rallies Won	% Rallies won at the net
	% 1st Serve points won	% 1st Serve points won serving to deuce court
Rugby union	% of Tackles completed	% of Tackles (Type) completed in amber zone
	Number of Phases	% of Phases in red zone leading to points
	% Lineouts won	% 5 Man lineouts won in green zone
Netball	Number of centre passes	% Centre passes leading to goal
	% Shot accuracy	% Shot success per location
	% Possession Won	% Live turnover won in mid-court

In this situation as centre pass to goal play was quicker, a greater number of centre passes were played within the allocated time. While such assumptions can be useful to performance reviews, the aim of performance analysis is to provide objective and meaningful data.

Even with focused KPIs presented in Table 3.2, further consideration must be provided to definitions of both the indicators and the variables involved prior to commencing data collection. Focusing on the KPIs related to soccer, the analyst must consider the location of the final third entry; where does this area begin? How will it be accurately analysed? How will it be defined? Without clear parameters, location data in particular can become subjective to collect. Consider the view from the analyst station or angle of the camera recording the footage, are these in line with the entry area? Is the view distorted? Can markers on the pitch side be used to support the collection of location data? The final third entry metric, as supported by FIFA (2023), is an opportunity to gain insights into a team's attacking strengths and strategies. Based on the Premier League, soccer pitches are commonly 105 metres (Premier League, 2023) meaning the attacking third area would commence 35 metres from the opposing goal line. Yet, even once definitions are developed, a plan must be established to enable the accurate collection of data. Without marking the area 35 metres from the goal line, how will an analyst successfully recognise an entry in this zone?

A similar critical approach can also be applied to the netball and tennis performance indicators (Table 3.2). Firstly, evaluating the KPIs for tennis and to ensure consistency in the data collection process, it is advised that clear guidelines defining court boundaries are provided. A contentious example in tennis is the % of net points won, a statistic commonly seen in Grand Slam tennis tournaments (Wimbledon, 2023). Yet, where does this area begin and end? And how can this be defined? Is it as simple as playing a shot in the upper half of the court within the service box which is 6.4 metres from the net? In this instance and contrary to the final third in soccer example, court markings are available which can assist with the consistency of data collection.

Onto netball and the explanation of the KPI related to centre pass success (% Centre passes leading to goal). In some instances, this metric will focus on the success of centre passes leading directly to goal, meaning once the ball has been turned over, collection of data to that metric ceases (i.e., 0/1 Direct Centre Pass to Goal). On other occasions and dependent on coach and athlete needs, this metric may also investigate the entire centre pass sequence regardless of whether the ball has been turned over or not. Consider the occasion where Team A have a centre pass and Team B turnover the ball in the centre third from a live interception. On entering the shooting circle, the umpire calls an attacking player offside. This donates the ball back to Team A, who go onto score a goal. In terms of the overall centre pass sequence, Team A had the centre pass and scored from it (i.e., 1/1 Overall Centre Pass to Goal). It would also be noted in Team A's indicators that this score was not

Table 3.3 A summary KPIs related to centre passes in netball

Team A	*Key Performance Indicators*	*Team B*
1/1 = 100%	Overall Centre pass to goal	–
0/1 = 0%	Direct Centre pass to goal	–
1/1 = 100%	Gained possession to goal	0/1 = 0%

a direct centre pass to goal as possession was originally lost. Team B would be noted with a gained possession (live turnover) although this was not scored and Team A would also be noted with a gained possession (restart turnover) which was positively scored (see Table 3.3). Overall, the variation of KPIs relating to the performance of the centre pass provides a complete overview of the event and its outcomes.

Gathering meaningful data

To support analysts in developing data collection methods, Lemmick and Frencken (2013) discussed that four questions can be considered when reviewing an event, thus providing an accurate record of the actions taking place. These are:

What? How? Where? and **When?**

O'Donoghue (2015) additionally suggested that two further questions should be incorportaed to provide greater context and detail.

Who? and **Why**?

A model encompassing the six questions is presented in Figure 3.2. The model explains the connection between performance indicators and variables, and how it can be used when considering **'What to analyse'**?

The purpose of the model is to demonstrate the association between performance variables and indicators. A performance indicator is a combination

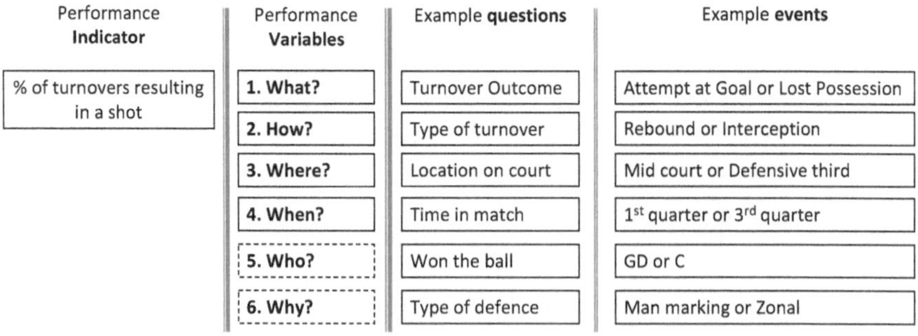

Figure 3.2 Six-step model, developed to gather quality information on sports performances.

of variables used to assess performance in match play and training (Hughes and Bartlett, 2002). A performance variable also known as action variable, is the raw event data required to generate the performance indicator. This can be measured on a series of scales, including nominal, ordinal, ratio and interval. In relation to Figure 3.2, the scales of data have been assigned below:

Nominal:

- Location on court (defensive, mid or attacking third)
- Who won the ball (GK, GD, WD, C, WA, GA, GS)

Ordinal:

- Turnover outcome (attempt at goal or loss of possession)

Interval/Ratio:

- % of turnovers resulting in a shot
- one attacking rebound from three attempts

Operating the model

It is important to operate the model from left to right; firstly, identifying the KPI you wish to gather. Using the six variables and example questions, consider what details are important to calculate the KPI? In this case, we firstly need to establish an outcome to the turnover. Did the team successfully transition the ball from the turnover to a shot at goal? If not, an assumption is that the opposition successfully regained the ball. Simply in this case, Team A turn over the ball but lost possession prior to attempting a shot at goal, therefore, one turnover > one loss possession = 0% of turnovers resulting in a shot.

Whilst the KPI does not explicitly request details on type of turnover, location of turnover or time in match, this information will add quality to data collection. Figure 3.3 presents an additional but not an exhaustive list of KPIs that can be calculated by gathering information using the six-step model above. At this stage, it must be stated that KPIs are a combination of variables (Hughes and Bartlett, 2002), this is not exclusively a combination of two variables. Below is an example of combining three action variables, but note it can be greater than three.

Example of combining three action variables

% of live turnovers to shot in quarter 4 is an example of combining three action variables to meet its criteria. Building on the example above, hypothetically Team A turn over the ball through an interception by a player in the fourth quarter. On this occasion, the ball is successfully transitioned

Performance **Indicator**	Performance **Variables**	Example **questions**	Example **events**
% of turnovers resulting in a shot	1. What?	Turnover Outcome	Attempt at Goal or Lost Possession
	2. How?	Type of turnover	Rebound or Interception
% of defensive rebounds in quarter 1	3. Where?	Location on court	Mid court or Defensive third
% of mid-court turnovers in quarter 2	4. When?	Time in match	1st quarter or 3rd quarter
	5. Who?	Won the ball	GD or C
% of live turnovers to shot in quarter 4	6. Why?	Type of defence	Man marking or Zonal

Explained:

% of live turnovers to shot in quarter 4	How?	Interception
	What?	Attempt at Goal
	When?	4th Quarter

Figure 3.3 Six-step model presenting and explaining the array of KPIs that can be calculated.

to the shooting circle whereby the GS (goal shooter) scores a goal. From an analysis perspective, this is one live turnover (*How*) + quarter four (*When*) + shot (*What*) = 100% successful of live turnovers to shot in quarter four.

It is here that we have a further opportunity to link back to *standard*? By allocating a reference to *when (time periods in netball), it creates an opportunity to draw comparisons between performances in other quarters of the match.

What it takes to win

The gathering of accurate information is one role of the performance analyst. The confirmation of KPIs, the definition of terms, the development of data collection systems, piloting of methods and the check for reliability are all steps taken prior to the collection of any data (see Chapters 4 and 5). Yet post data collection, the focus turns to the presentation of KPIs and feedback of information to athletes and coaches (see Chapter 8). These are the recipients of the information, and therefore the presentation of results must be clear and informative about the performance and what is required to win. With quality and detailed objective information, a true reflection of performance can be provided. For instance, data may highlight that performance was excellent in periods, whilst then equally focusing attention towards areas that were not. Objective data is influential when used correctly; if quality and detail is incorporated then an abundance of questions can be asked to investigate scenarios where performance was good or poor, ensuring the users of the information are best informed of the next steps, in what it takes to win (WITTW).

Yet, support around an athlete or team is not solely a performance analyst gathering video and objective data. An example of a multidisciplinary team is the UKSI. Here, the team behind the team, comprises of experts in strength and conditioning, physiology, nutrition, biomechanics, lifestyle, physiotherapy, psychology as well as performance analysts, all supporting elite athletes in a bid to perform at the highest level. The specialists bring a wide range of expertise enabling a strategy to impact performance and in the case of UKSI, led by a head of service who oversees the provision connecting science, medicine and technology (UK Sports Institute, 2023). A similar infrastructure is also noted in academy soccer (Raya-Castellano and Uriondo, 2015), and with a range of sport science roles advertised in elite level soccer, a similar framework is assumed. To aid explanations a simulated infrastructure illustrating the alignment of roles can be seen in Figure 3.4. Each discipline has been categorised into one of three areas: Mind, Body and Technology, and whilst disciplines are stacked, they hold no hierarchical power over another. The purpose of the figure alone is to demonstrate the shared focus of each area, for example, physiology and strength and conditioning are both relating

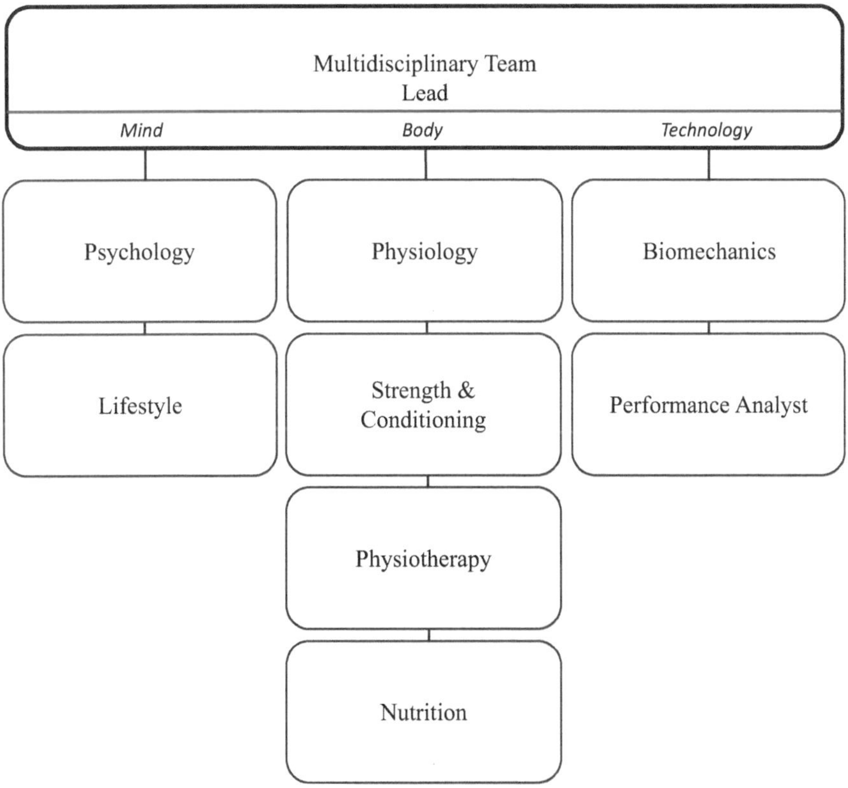

Figure 3.4 A simulated multidisciplinary team infrastructure to demonstrate a connection between roles.

to the body of the performer. In this sense, a close working relationship between these practitioners would be expected to ensure the athlete is best prepared. It would also be naive to assume that each discipline is set to these individual categories; within sport these disciplines will naturally overlap to support the athlete. As an example, consider how a performance analyst can support an athlete returning to play post injury. Firstly, the practitioner may be involved in providing footage of the injury to support rehabilitation (Body) whist later supporting the psychologist (Mind) with video sequences of positive performances or footage of latest training sessions to ensure they are ready to return.

Of course, at times, specialist practitioners will operate independently with athletes, yet a holistic method whereby support staff share values and collaboratively work together is deemed a more favourable approach. In doing so, the support team share a collective responsibility for the athlete's or team's performance. The availability of specialised support staff is of course a privilege and most common at elite level sport, and even in these cases, provision may be organised in a way that discipline staff rarely cross paths as a result of session demands, training schedules or budgets preventing staff to be full time practitioners. In this case, communication between disciplines is deemed an even higher priority.

The implementation of a multidisciplinary team to support the development of an athlete or team is key. It requires an environment whereby discipline experts are well-connected to each other, sharing similar values to enable an athlete or team to perform at the highest level.

Conclusions

One role of the performance analyst is to provide reliable and meaningful data to the performer and their coach. In doing so, it is important that quality information is provided that supports the coaching process and aligns to the values of the recipients of feedback. To support the generation of valuable data, the six-step model comprising of six questions (Figure 3.2) can be implemented. The model demonstrates an ability to combine two or more variables, in the generation of detailed key performance indicators. Taking a wider perspective, it is also important to reflect on the role of the performance analyst in a multidisciplinary team. The WITTW approach specifically draws together sport science experts to work collaboratively in supporting high performance athletes. In this instance, the performance analyst has the capacity to share meaningful data freely with other discipline experts of the multidisciplinary team, in an approach to support the development of athletes and teams.

4 Manual notation systems

Introduction

This chapter will explore manual notation systems and their relevance in analysing sports performance. Details of how to design a manual notation system and what a performance analyst must consider in this process, from input to output, will also be covered.

Why use manual notation systems?

With an abundance of computerised analysis systems available in industry, which are becoming more cost-effective approaches to evaluate performance (see Chapter 6), many may rightly question the need and use for manual hand notation methods when they fail to combine match statistics with video sequences. The combination of objective data and video clips is a powerful evaluation tool to enhance performance and decision making in sport. Data providing information on what has happened, supplemented with video which provides context on the situation and an explanation on how the event occurred. So, when this partnership is lacking, why are we still considering the use of manual hand notation methods?

Contrary to the question above, we must first acknowledge the practice of computerised analysis packages and available software. Catering for the consumer and their analysis needs, providers such as HUDL SportsCode (HUDL, Lincoln, NE) and Nacsport (Nacsport, Gran Canaria, Spain) offer access to a range of software levels. These are organised on a spectrum and determined by the accessibility to features (see Chapter 5). Ranging from entry to professional level access (i.e., Nacsport Basic – Nacsport Elite), analysts have the freedom to purchase a package based on their personal workflow, provision needs and budget. Stepping away from the obligation of having to purchase a high-end *'one-size fits all'* range, which will come at an increased cost and with unwanted features, depending on analyst requirements and experience. In short, this method supports the accessibility of analysis resources for all, a provision which previously was marketed to professional and high-end consumers. Aside from software, an element often overlooked

DOI: 10.4324/9781003375463-4

when budgeting for analysis workstations is the consideration of hardware to operate the specialised performance analysis packages. Regardless of analysis aims (e.g. technical or technique), each package will provide information on recommended hardware requirements which includes details of RAM (random access memory) and processor units. Should you wish to capture footage live during a game or stream video, the requests are likely to require a higher-specification machine which naturally comes at a greater cost. Now having briefly touched upon capturing footage, there is also the consideration of purchasing a video camera and capturing devices to connect a video feed into a laptop or analyst's workstation. So, whilst computerised performance analysis packages are becoming more affordable, it is important to be mindful that software is not the sole cost.

Using information above, the role of manual notation systems is simple. It provides an entry level approach to analyse performances in competition or training environments, without the need or expense of software or hardware systems. Yes, a limitation is its restricted ability to neatly combine objective data and video sequences of observed performances, but it is a basic approach for gathering objective data and is a stepping stone to computerised platforms. Manual notation systems developed either on paper or on a computerised spreadsheet package have some worth; it's these progressions that will develop an analyst's knowledge and understanding of the performance analysis process. By stripping the process back to its inception, it allows users to understand the important aspects of performance, how to operationalise these and how to identify performance variables to generate selected key performance indicators (KPIs) (see Chapter 3). It is skills like this that can develop an aspiring performance analyst, not only to collect data but to have a true understanding of system development and the intricacies of how it operates.

Manual notation system design is not as simple as it may sound. Firstly, the system must meet the needs of the analysis; what type of data and KPIs are required? Secondly, you must consider when the coach requires the information; during or after performance? Simply by having a focus on what is required, a draft system can be initiated. Yet, it would be naive to think that system development ceases after draft one. Pilot testing ensures the method is valid and that the system meets the aims of analysis. This procedure involves the designing and redesigning of a system from input to output (discussed below) until it is fully operational to meet its aims. Whilst this procedure will need to be conducted for both manual and computerised packages, the development of these systems on paper or on a spreadsheet package provides the user with freedom to design and redesign in any location and without hardware or software constraints. This could include, live at a training session, in the match environment, or by using pre-recorded footage of a performance that has already taken place.

As a whole, some manual notation systems provide immediate feedback for users and the objective data collected can inform coaching decisions and impact performance (O'Donoghue, 2015: 106–112). Even without linked video sequences, manual notation systems are invaluable and can reinforce coach observations, this is particularly important when considering experienced coaches only accurately recall 59.2% of events during 45 minutes of a football match (Laird and Waters, 2008). In this situation and without performance analysis support, consider the effectiveness of half-time feedback? Therefore, whilst not as streamlined as computerised systems in combining objective data and video sequences, manual approaches are certainly valuable. They provide aspiring performance analysts with an understanding of system development whilst outwardly influencing feedback messages to performers who previously relied solely on the subjective observations of coaches.

Manual hand notation systems

Hughes and Franks (2004) described three types of manual notation systems which can be used in isolation or in partnership with another. These approaches are:

1 Sequential
2 Frequency
3 Scatter

Below, using **Input**, **Throughput** and **Output** which relates to the phases of an analysis process, each approach is explained in detail. First, system design and collection of data; second, the generation of KPIs and third, the presentation of results gathered using manual notation methods. Regardless of the approach selected, progression through each phase is still required, albeit time spent in each phase will differ. This will become clearer in later sections.

Input

Input is the process that involves the gathering of data. Firstly, this must begin by having an understanding of the aims of the analysis (type of data and KPIs required). This will naturally aid the decision of which manual notation system to choose. Once a system has been confirmed, defining selected KPIs and confirming the action variables to collect is needed. As its name suggests, input proposes 'the inputting of data', yet the phase also includes the work in preparation for this step. Prior to collecting any data, operational definitions and terminology of events must be confirmed; this is to support consistency and accuracy of data collection. A reliability task must be completed whether there is a sole or a group of analysts. For a sole analyst, its purpose is for consistency and accuracy (i.e. recording a certain tackle type in rugby consistently throughout the match). For a group of analysts, this task is important to confirm that there is a shared understanding of actions (i.e. two or more analysts labelling certain tackle types accurately across a number of fixtures). Shared language and an understanding of terminology is important when analysing performance, whether that be a shared understanding between analysts or equally important a shared understanding between analysts and the recipients of the information (the athletes and coaches). In the development of relationships with coaches, definitions and terminology can be checked and challenged. It would be naive to assume that definitions of action variables or KPIs are consistent between individuals, so it is always important to (re-)confirm. Depending on the coach's preference or the complexity of the action, a video catalogue of actions may be preferred over a written description. With either approach, the resource can be shared with partners prior to a meeting to clarify definitions.

Each system with respect to the input phase is described below.

Input: sequential systems

A **sequential** system is a detailed and methodical approach to analysing performance. The system gathers event data in chronological order which allows for the patterns of performance to be determined. Depending on the focus of analysis, each entry can be described based on a number of variables. This can include, game period, location of event, player involved, type of event and outcome.

Example 1: Tennis

Figure 4.1 is an extract of a sequential analysis system used to evaluate the effectiveness of the tennis serve and its association with rally outcome. Data entries are recorded in rows yet described against action variables listed in columns. In this case, reading from left to right, each serve has 11 descriptive labels from set to score. Whilst no doubt the sequential system holds more detail over its alternatives (frequency tables and scatter diagrams), it does come with its limitations. Unlike other approaches, data collected using a sequential system is not ready to be presented to coaches

Set	Service Game	Server	Serve	Serve Location	Serve Zone	Serve Outcome	Rally Outcome	End Shot Type	End Shot Location	Score
1	1	Player 1	1st	Deuce	Wide	In	Player 1 Won	Backhand Drive	Zone 3	15 - 0
1	1	Player 1	1st	Advantage	Wide	Fault	N/A	N/A	N/A	15 - 0
1	1	Player 1	2nd	Advantage	T	In	Player 2 Won	Backhand Drive	Zone 3	15 - 15
1	1	Player 1	1st	Deuce	Wide	Fault	N/A	N/A	N/A	15 - 15
1	1	Player 1	2nd	Deuce	Body	In	Player 1 Won	Backhand X Drive	Zone 3	30 - 15
1	1	Player 1	1st	Advantage	Wide	Fault	N/A	N/A	N/A	30 - 15
1	1	Player 1	2nd	Advantage	T	In	Player 1 Won	Forehand Drop	Zone 2	40 - 15
1	1	Player 1	1st	Deuce	Wide	Fault	N/A	N/A	N/A	40 - 15
1	1	Player 1	2nd	Deuce	Body	In	Player 2 Won	Forehand Drive	Zone 4	40 - 30
1	1	Player 1	1st	Advantage	Wide	In	Player 2 Won	Backhand X Drive	Zone 3	Deuce
1	1	Player 1	1st	Deuce	Wide	Fault	N/A	N/A	N/A	Deuce
1	1	Player 1	2nd	Deuce	Body	In	Player 1 Won	Backhand Drive	Zone 3	Adv. Player 1
1	1	Player 1	1st	Advantage	Body	Fault	N/A	N/A	N/A	Adv. Player 1
1	1	Player 1	2nd	Advantage	Body	In	Player 2 Won	Backhand X Drive	Zone 3	Deuce
1	1	Player 1	1st	Deuce	Wide	In	Player 1 Won	Backhand Drop	Zone 1	Adv. Player 1
1	1	Player 1	1st	Advantage	T	In	Player 1 Won	Forehand Drive	Zone 4	Game

Figure 4.1 An example of a sequential system used to gather data on the tennis serve and the rally outcome.

immediately post-performance. This is due to the inclusion of several variables, the quantity of data collected and the frequencies not already being cross-tabulated. Therefore, a further data processing procedure is required to combine performance variables and generate the KPIs used to measure performance. As an example, Figure 4.1 presents data collected from one game of tennis. Consider the quantity of information for one set and later an entire match and trying to make sense of the information without further processing! The aim of the analysis presented in Figure 4.1 is to explore the effectiveness of the tennis service, not only focusing on the initial location (advantage or deuce court) but specifically the zone within that area (T, body, wide). Whilst the serve outcome can be noted, further data is then collected on the rally outcome and includes shot type and location of shot. The depth of information presents an opportunity for end users to develop and determine patterns of performance. Within the aims of analysis, a list of KPIs (not exhaustive) includes: percentage of first serve in, percentage of first serve points won, percentage of first serves to the advantage court won and percentage of first serves to the advantage court (wide zone) won.

Example 2: Boxing

All input systems are blank canvases, and so sequential systems can be developed to evaluate other sports types such as combat, cyclic sports and technique intensive actions. Using boxing as an example, Figure 4.2 presents a blank sequential system for analysis of a boxing bout. This system can be used to analyse the performance of one or two performers simultaneously, although it is more difficult to accurately collect data if completed for both performers in live event. This simple sequential system allows the analyst to conduct an investigation into punches thrown in a boxing match. The action variables include type of punch, whether contact was made to the opponent (and if so, where) and lastly the location of where the boxer was standing in the ring during this period. Whether separated per round or presented for the overall fight, the KPIs for the investigation are: the percentage of overall punches landed, percentage of each punch type landed, distribution of punches by contact location, percentage of shot landed in the centre of ring and on the ropes. Further variables can also be combined to generate more specific KPIs. These include the percentage of jab punches landed to the head.

Boxer	Round	Punch Type	Landed (Y/N)	Combination Punch	Contact Location	Ring Location

Figure 4.2 A blank sequential system to evaluate punches thrown in a boxing bout.

Over	Ball	Line & Length	Delivery Type	Bowler Type	Runs
1	1	Full Straight	Stock	Right Arm Medium	1
1	2	Good Off Side	Leg Cutter	Right Arm Medium	0
1	3	Good Straight	Leg Cutter	Right Arm Medium	3
1	4	Good Straight	Off Cutter	Right Arm Medium	0
1	5	Short Off Side	Slower Ball	Right Arm Medium	0
1	6	Good Straight	Off Cutter	Right Arm Medium	0

Figure 4.3 An extract of data collected using a sequential system on bowling performance in cricket.

Example 3: Cricket

Figure 4.3 presents an extract of data collected from an over in a cricket match. This system aims to evaluate the performance of a bowler, demonstrating that a sequential system can also be used to evaluate technique type actions. In this case, by gathering data per ball and over an opportunity is presented to explore whether any bowling strategies are used during particular periods of the match. As well as delivery types, the number of runs is also included, giving an evaluation of run rate, dot balls and wickets taken per bowler.

Data validation

To enhance data collection using a sequential system and limit user error on data entry, it is advised to add data validation to each performance variable column. This approach not only reduces data entry errors with respect to inputting information (e.g. incorrect spelling of actions or spaces accidentally placed after the word) but also increases the speed of data entry. This is a useful strategy, when collecting data in live event. Whilst the initial example of data entry errors (spelling and spacing) may not seem as an inconvenience during data collection, it certainly does become an inconvenience during the throughput process. Data entry errors, as seen in Table 4.1, result in the same action being recognised in two or three formats, mainly based on its spelling or its structure. In essence, Table 4.1 should present advantage and deuce court locations once in the first column with frequencies of their occurrences split between serving zones (wide, body, T). In this case, advantage is listed as three different values. To the naked eye, there is no difference between

Table 4.1 Example of a pivot table

Count of Serve Zone	**Column Labels**			
Row Labels	**Body**	**T**	**Wide**	**Grand Total**
Advantage	2	3	1	6
Advantage			1	1
Advantge			1	1
Deuce	3		5	8
Grand Total	**5**	**3**	**8**	**16**

its presentation in row one and two, unlike the case in row three where the entry is clearly spelt incorrectly. Although row two is spelt the same, a space is present at the end of the word. Structurally, this then appears different and is placed in a separate row within the pivot table. This can be resolved by locating the event on the data collection sheet and simply updating, which may take some time as they look the same. A quicker resolution would be to use the find and replace function within the spreadsheet package.

Data validation setup

To overcome the issues raised above and to create an efficient sequential system workflow, data validation is recommended. Within the Excel data collection workbook, set up a worksheet solely named 'Data Validation Options' and copy across the column headings from the sequential system created (Figure 4.4).

It is important here to identify all possible options that may occur under each variable heading, for example: Set 1, 2, 3, 4 and 5. Whilst the match selected for analysis might be completed in three sets, it is useful to have a complete system design that can be transferred to evaluate future performances. The pilot test can also support this phase, particularly when validating the system. On the spot, it may seem that all variable options have been listed, yet by observing footage to assess the system prior to commencing data collection, further event types might be raised, i.e., a tie breaker in tennis. This event occurs occasionally and would need to be listed under service game.

Once all variable options have been listed under relevant headings, data validation can be set up in the data collection worksheet. This must be completed independently for each column. Within the **Data collection** worksheet, highlight the first column for as many rows as you require. In this example, data validation will be set up to row 50. Once highlighted, select **Data** and **Data Validation**. In a new window, select **List** in the allow text box and within **Source** navigate to the '**Data Validation Options**' worksheet. Here, select the data options relevant to that variable and column (see Figure 4.5 column A) and press OK to confirm. Drop-down lists will now be available in column A of the **Data collection** worksheet, up to row 50. Repeat the process for the remainder of the worksheet and columns.

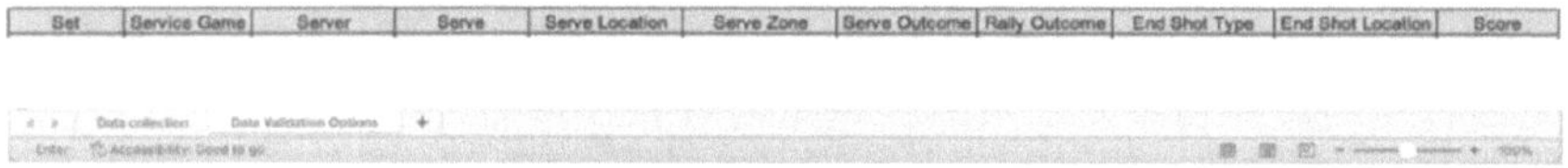

Figure 4.4 A worksheet setup for data validation, whereby all variable options must be listed under column headings.

A	B	C	D	E	F
Set	**Service Game**	**Server**	**Serve**	**Serve Location 1**	**Serve Zone**
1	1	Player 1	1st	Deuce	Wide
2	2	Player 2	2nd	Advantage	Body
3	3				T
4	4				
5	5				
	6				
	7				
	8				
	9				
	10				
	11				
	12				
	Tie Break				

Figure 4.5 Illustrating the setup of data validation lists and the inclusion of all variable options.

Input: frequency tables

A **frequency table** is a quick and convenient method to gather objective data on performance. A frequency table can be created on a computer package or written up on paper. The former provides the opportunity to print multiple copies for use in future matches, whilst the latter would need replicating or redrawing. Whilst the development of a frequency table would look more aesthetically pleasing if made electronically, it is far more convenient to collect data by pen and paper. A frequency table collects information using tallies, essentially noting a mark in a cell when an event occurs. This approach can be conducted live during fixtures or at training sessions, with feedback immediately available for athletes and coaches. A limitation of the frequency table is the ability to collect information in chronological order and whilst new tables can be used for each quarter, half or game; it would be impossible to determine which event occurred first within those periods. As with all manual notation methods, systems can be developed for any aspect of performance in most sports. Following guidelines, blank canvases can be transformed by performance analysts to gather information on a sport of choice. An example of a frequency table for use in netball can be seen in Figure 4.6.

Figure 4.6 provides an opportunity to collect objective data in netball focusing on the origin of possession and their success. This is an example that can easily be modified for other possession based sports. KPIs of focus in this example are the percentage of centre passes that result in a goal (success) and percentage of interception success. This can be done for both teams as shown in Figure 4.7. The table is simple to use; first, you must note a tally in the origin of possession column, in short how possession started. It is then important to observe performance and note if that sequence ended in a goal. If not and the ball was turned over, a new origin of possession tally would be noted in the opposition team column. This procedure then continues for each quarter.

Team 1			Team 2	
Scored	Count	Origin/Indicator	Count	Scored
		Centre Pass		
		Interception		
		Outline (sideline)		
		Backline		
		Toss up		
		Defensive Rebound		
		Free/Penalty		
		Total		

Figure 4.6 Example of a frequency table for use in netball.

<table>
<tr><th colspan="2">Team 1</th><th></th><th colspan="2">Team 2</th></tr>
<tr><td>Scored</td><td>Count</td><td>Origin/Indicator</td><td>Count</td><td>Scored</td></tr>
<tr><td>||</td><td>||||</td><td>Centre Pass</td><td>||||</td><td>||||</td></tr>
<tr><td></td><td></td><td>Interception</td><td>||</td><td>|</td></tr>
<tr><td></td><td></td><td>Outline (sideline)</td><td></td><td></td></tr>
<tr><td></td><td></td><td>Backline</td><td></td><td></td></tr>
<tr><td></td><td></td><td>Toss up</td><td></td><td></td></tr>
<tr><td></td><td></td><td>Defensive Rebound</td><td></td><td></td></tr>
<tr><td></td><td></td><td>Free/Penalty</td><td></td><td></td></tr>
<tr><td></td><td></td><td>Total</td><td></td><td></td></tr>
</table>

Figure 4.7 An extract on data collection in netball using a frequency table.

In comparison to the sequential system, event data collected using a frequency table is less detailed. As an example, Figure 4.7 fails to include information relating to court location, player involvement or turnover types. Yet, the strength of a frequency table is its ability to impact performance immediately. Data gathered using this method can be calculated and presented to coaches and athletes during the performances or immediately after. This is an advantage it holds over the sequential system, which as we're aware requires further data processing before having the ability to communicate results.

Input: scatter diagrams

A **scatter diagram** is the most visual method of the three manual notation systems. This approach uses a diagram related to the sport to collect data. This could be the whole pitch or court area, or if analysis was focused on a specific zone, then a diagram representing this area could alternatively be used. In soccer, this could be half a pitch to gather data on shooting locations. Scatter diagrams are versatile and can also be used to collect data on combat sports or record a sequence of movement patterns. A diagram could be used to plot a gymnastics floor routine, dance performance or even map where contact was made during a boxing bout. The latter has opportunities to use

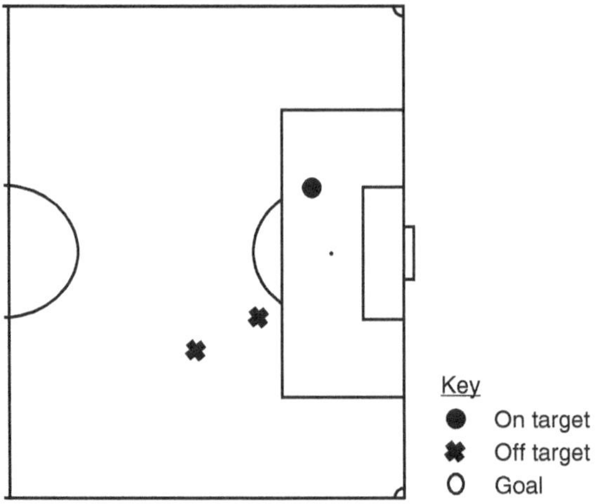

Figure 4.8 An example of a scatter diagram used to collect shot locations in soccer.

either a boxing ring to map fighting locations or an outline of a boxer to plot where contact was made to the body.

Figure 4.8 is an example from soccer, whereby shapes have been used to dictate the outcome of the event (shots in this case) from specific locations on the pitch. A strength of this approach is the ability to conduct analysis live either during performances or at training. The collection of information on a map provides a clear visual representation of events without the need to process data further before feeding back to performers and coaches. Whilst, in its simple format, the order of events may not be established, this could simply be overcome by noting numbers next to each shape when entering data. A limitation of this method is the brief level of information gathered on the aspect of performance. Take Figure 4.8 as an example, whilst the location and the outcome of the shot are noted, details relating to how the ball was received in that area are omitted. Things to consider: where the ball came from - set piece or open play? The player who passed the ball? The player who took the shot? and the type of shot? It is fair to say that the scatter diagram holds its place in gathering objective data on performances, should you require quick and basic information. Yet, for more detailed information, its use would be best combined with the frequency or sequential system.

Figure 4.9 is an example of combining the scatter diagram with a sequential system. This combination allows the analyst to draw on the benefits of using a comprehensive data collection method alongside the visual presentation of data, that the scatter diagram provides. Figure 4.9 is an example used in a squash doubles match, whereby two athletes (Player A and B) battle an opposing team. In this example, the analysis focuses on the rally end outcome with particular attention on shot type and location on court where the shot was played. Using the principles of the sequential system, data for each rally is entered from left to right. Alongside the sequential system, a scatter diagram

Game	Player	Team	Name	Outcome	Shot Type	Area	Score
1	Player A	Team 1	Error	Error	Volley Short	11	00:01
1	Player B	Team 2	Winner	Let	X Lob	5	00:02
1	Player A	Team 2	Winner	Winner	Serve	9	00:02
1	Player B	Team 1	Winner	Winner	Volley Drop	9	01:02
1	Player B	Team 2	Error	Error	Drive	13	02:02
1	Player A	Team 2	Error	Error	Volley Boast	12	03:02
1	Player B	Team 2	Error	Error	Boast	13	04:02

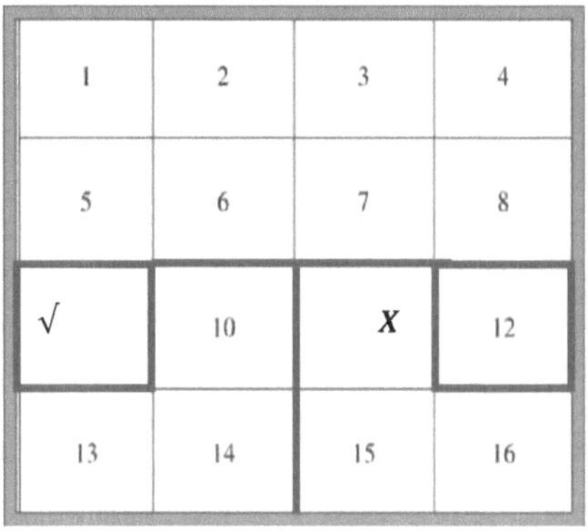

Figure 4.9 An example where two input methods have been combined (sequential and scatter) to analyse a doubles squash match.

of a squash court has been constructed with 16 zones, each zone representing a location on the court. Using data for Team 1, symbols have been allocated to the diagram demonstrating where winners and errors were made during the first game. This gives an instant visual representation of where rallies are won or lost. It is also important to note the rally end zone in the sequential system, this provides a link between the two approaches and will allow end users to identify patterns between results. In this example, it could be between shot type and court location, or shot type and outcome.

A limitation of scatter diagrams is the accumulation of events per diagram and its ability to become quickly congested. Depending on the aims of the analysis, be mindful that a new scatter diagram may be required per game, per round or per half, depending on sport, which will allow data to be easily interpreted and also patterns between events in set time periods to also be established.

Throughput

Throughput is the process that refers to the generation of KPIs from raw data collected using the selected manual notation systems discussed above. Regardless of manual notation system (sequential, frequency or scatter), this step would need to be completed to normalise the data. The depth of processing, however, would depend on which input method was used. In short, raw data collected using an input system should not be presented to coaches and athletes without being processed.

Throughput: sequential systems

A strength of the sequential system is the ability to collect detailed data on performances, yet we are aware that this poses a limitation with data processing. As this method is the most comprehensive of the three approaches, the depth of the throughput process is also the greatest. Post-data collection and using the aims and objectives of the analysis, pivot tables can be assembled to combine performance variables in rows and columns to generate the required performance indicators. To create a pivot table, highlight all entries in the data collection worksheet including column headings, then select the **Insert** tab and select **Pivot Table**. By highlighting data in advance, a green border will appear around the data and the correct cell references will appear in the **range** text box of the new window. For ease, position the pivot table in a new worksheet and rename the tab once set-up. Initially, the pivot table will appear blank with a **PivotTable Fields** window appearing on the right-hand side of the page. A reason for highlighting column headings alongside the data when initially setting up the pivot table should now become apparent, as column heading names will appear in the **Field Name box.**

Using column heading names, which also serve as variable headings, select and drag the required titles into column and row boxes (step one). Step two, drag a duplicate of a previously selected variable into the values box. In short, step one will create the table whilst step two will populate the table with results. Some confusion may arise when selecting what variables to place in columns and rows? Here, it must be noted that it does not matter in terms of generating results as the information will be same, and the only difference is its appearance. See Figure 4.10a; we have placed **Outcome** into the columns text box and **Serve** into rows. Data in the corresponding pivot table aligns to this with 1st and 2nd serve data listed in rows 3 and 4, respectively. In Figure 4.10b, we have swapped the location of these variables (column – serve; row – outcome). In rows 3–5, rally outcome data (fault, lost, won) will now be presented. Referring to Figures 4.10a and 4.10b, you will recognise the results are the same regardless of the construction of the pivot table.

(a)

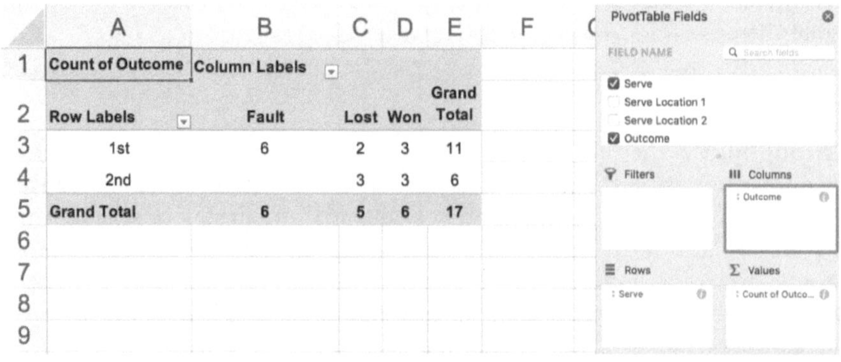

Figure 4.10 (a) Illustrating the approaches to setting up a pivot table. *(Continued)*

(b)

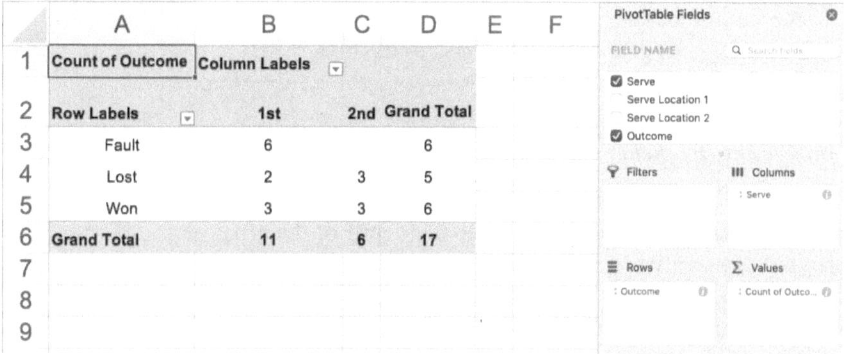

	A	B	C	D	E	F
1	Count of Outcome	Column Labels				
2	Row Labels	1st	2nd	Grand Total		
3	Fault	6		6		
4	Lost	2	3	5		
5	Won	3	3	6		
6	Grand Total	11	6	17		
7						
8						
9						

Figure 4.10 *(Continued)* (b) Illustrating the approaches to setting up a pivot table.

Once the data have been cross-tabulated using the pivot table, results can be generated for each key performance indicator. Using Figure 4.10a and concentrating on the KPI of % of rallies won on the second serve, the following steps can be followed to produce a result:

KPI:	% of rallies won on the second serve
Variables required:	Number of second serves (cell E4) Number of rallies won on a second serve (cell D4)
Equation:	= (D4: number of rallies won / E4: number of serves)*100 = (3/6)*100 = **50%** of rallies won on the second serve.

Using the list of KPIs identified within the aims of the investigation, further calculations can be conducted by updating the combination of variables in the column and row fields of the pivot table. Once cross-tabulated, follow the steps above to normalise results. Note that KPIs are a combination of two or more variables, so adding additional variables into field boxes is recommended. See Figure 4.11 which combines service number, serve location and rally outcome, which will generate the selection of KPIs listed below:

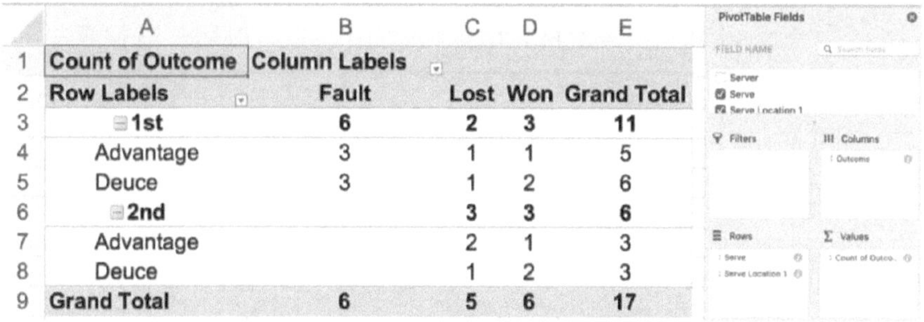

	A	B	C	D	E
1	Count of Outcome	Column Labels			
2	Row Labels	Fault	Lost	Won	Grand Total
3	1st	6	2	3	11
4	Advantage	3	1	1	5
5	Deuce	3	1	2	6
6	2nd		3	3	6
7	Advantage		2	1	3
8	Deuce		1	2	3
9	Grand Total	6	5	6	17

Figure 4.11 Presentation of a pivot table with multiple variables selected to generate detailed KPI results.

- Percentage of first and second serves in
- Percentage of first and second serve points won
- Percentage of first and second serves to the advantage court won
- Percentage of first and second serves to the deuce court won

Throughput: frequency tables

The throughput process for the frequency table is far more straightforward than the sequential system procedure, yet the depth of data may not allow for patterns to be as easily identified. Using raw data collected in netball (Figure 4.12), the following steps will explain how to generate KPIs using data collected in a frequency table.

Team 1			**Team 2**	
Scored	Count	Origin/Indicator	Count	Scored
2 II	4 IIII	Centre Pass	IIII 4	IIII 4
		Interception	II 2	I 1
		Outline (sideline)		
		Backline		
		Toss up		
		Defensive Rebound		
		Free/Penalty		
		Total		

Figure 4.12 An example of a frequency table used in netball with results totalled.

To begin, total the raw data tallied in the frequency table per indicator (Figure 4.12). Using count and success values, the KPIs for origin success can then be calculated. Focusing of the % of Centre Passes (CP) scored, results for both teams can be generated.

KPI:	% of Centre Passes scored
Variables required:	Number of CP (Team 1) Number of CP scored (Team 1)
Equation:	= (Number of CP scored / Number of CP)*100 = (2/4)*100 = **50%** of Team 1 centre passes result in a goal

In comparison to Team 1's performance, Team 2 reported to score four from four CPs, giving a 100% success rate of scoring from a centre pass. Team 2 also intercepted the ball on two occasions, but only scoring from one; this giving a 50% success rate of interceptions to goal. This a simple and effective approach to generate objective data which can inform the coaching process. Using this format, a quick comparison of results can be made across opposing teams, this is to identify the effectiveness of their CP attack or defensive strategies.

Throughput: scatter charts

The scatter chart requires the least amount of processing on completion of data collection, in comparison to the two other methods (sequential system and frequency table). Based on its visual nature, the image below could be presented to coaches and athletes immediately post-performance. Yet, to enhance its impact, some processing can be completed to provide objective data alongside its visual presentation. See Figure 4.13 whereby totals have been added for each category. Using this raw data, the KPI of % of shots on target can be generated.

KPI:	% of shots on target
Variables required:	Total number of shots Total number of shots on target
Equation:	= (Total number of shots on target / Total number of shots)*100 = (1/3)*100 = **33%** of shots on target.

Elaborating on this example, KPIs related to locations can also be calculated. Consider: % of shots on target inside the penalty area (1/1), % of shots on target outside the penalty area (0/2).

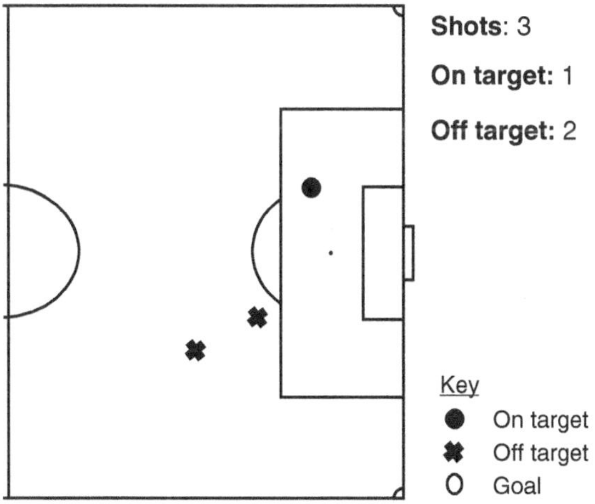

Figure 4.13 An example of processing data collected using a scatter diagram.

Output

Output refers to the presentation of KPIs generated from the throughput process and regardless of input method selected, the same guidance applies to this phase. It is essential that KPIs relate to the aims of the analysis or investigation and are presented clearly. Once the throughput process has been completed and the indicators set out to be generated have been calculated, our focus must move to how the information is presented for coaches and athletes.

Depending on environment (see Chapter 8), some outputs of analysis may be provided to athletes during performances, and so it is important that the information is clearly organised and is easy to understand in a short glance, ideally on one A4 page. Information presented must be meaningful to aid coaches with decision making and to help make impactful choices on the immediate next steps that can influence performance. Naturally, post-performance, it is likely that individuals involved will have more time to interpret and digest objective information and so outputs are likely to be more comprehensive, all in keeping with the principles of presenting information, which will be discussed below.

There are eight principles to consider when developing a one-page results dashboard for coaches and performers. These simple principles provide the analyst with a framework to aid the construction and presentation of their work. Whilst the input and throughput processes are related to the development of an analysis system and the generation of KPIs, which are unlikely to be seen by external stakeholders such as coaches and athletes. It is the output (dashboard in this case) which will communicate the work of the analyst and showcase results to an audience. To aid the development of this feedback vehicle, consider the following eight principles, seen in Table 4.2.

When developing a feedback resource, remember that the data is the most important feature. A dashboard feature or principle should not distract attention but instead be used to enhance and support information, enabling it to be quickly understood and digested. Should a dashboard need further explanation or if at first glance, attention is diverted, some adjustments should be made. Consider sharing your dashboard with others, their feedback can be valuable in the development of an effective feedback resource.

Conclusions

There are three manual notation systems available to gather objective data in sport. These are sequential systems, frequency tables and scatter diagrams. Using the phases input, throughput and output, comprehensive systems can be generated to gather objective data to support the coaching process. Each method does hold a collection of strengths and limitations; the sequential system is a detailed manual notation method. The vast data set allows for patterns to be drawn, albeit once a further data processing procedure has been conducted using pivot tables. Naturally, this process is time consuming

Table 4.2 Eight principles to consider when developing a manual notation output dashboard

Principle	*Description*
Invisibility	The dashboard has a clear design which focuses solely on the content. There are no distractions or conflicts that detract attention from the information in terms of colour, shapes or logos. Through good positioning, information can be easily interpreted by users with limited effort.
Scale	Use font size and formatting tools to highlight the most important information on the dashboard for coaches to see promptly. To draw attention to selected KPIs, increase the text size for it to stand out over other results.
Alignment	This can improve the presentation of information and ensure data presented is organised. Consider how a table can align results in rows and columns, which allow a coach to extract and compare results quickly.
Repetition	Repeat the presentation and format of results to emphasise a common theme. Information for opposing teams (home and away) or performers (player 1 and player 2) should be aligned, and KPIs repeated in a similar order for quick comparisons to be drawn.
Contrast	Use colour and shape to highlight contrasting results. As an example, this could be a red, amber, green (RAG) system whereby positive results are filled in green or results for a KPI which are below a target threshold may be filled in red.
Proximity	This refers to the positioning of information and the importance of keeping elements that belong together, together. As an example, information related to attack should be organised in one area of the dashboard, with KPIs relating to defence in another area.
Intuitive	An element in the dashboard should suggest its function without further description. For example, green suggests positive (go) and red suggests negative (stop). This can also refer to chart types, bar chart can show can show discrete comparisons, whereby a line chart suggests a trend.
Simplicity	Consider if all the data collected is required in a chart or table? Design of a dashboard can also relate to the use of white space or the simplifying of charts. For example, the removal of axis lines or filled chart background colours which may draw unwanted attention to that feature.

and so information cannot be immediately available for coaches. The frequency table can overcome this, with data processed almost immediately due to the format in which data is collected. The most visual method of the three manual notation systems is the scatter diagram. This system allows for precise location data to be recorded, a strength it holds over the other two approaches.

5 Developing a computerised system

Introduction

This chapter covers the use of manual video analysis software within sports performance analysis. Hugely versatile, manually operated systems can be tailored to develop systems that can support the collection, analysis and presentation of quantitative data and video sequences in sports of the user's choice. In an applied coaching context, users (i.e. analysts) are required to collect objective statistical data to inform visual feedback in the form of video sequences. For this purpose, analysts must develop robust data collection procedures (inputs), apply suitable software features to organise meta-data and video (throughputs) and employ effective mechanisms to share data and video (outputs). Although, the stages of system development for scientific research are similar to those in an applied coaching setting, scientific research systems are not often required to support interactive video feedback. Moving forward, the focus of the current chapter will be the development of systems for use in applied coaching contexts, readers interested in system development orientated towards research methods should see (O'Donoghue et al., 2012) for further assistance.

One of the first considerations when developing a manual computerised system is the need to identify the types of information and outputs required. Importantly, analysts should discuss the requirements of the system with coaching staff to establish what they want to see from the analysis. This may require considering performance indicators and working backwards to the variables (e.g. actions/events) that need to be input into the system. As an example, a coach may simply require the frequency (occurrence) of an action in a match, such as aerial duels in soccer. On the other hand, coaches may want to know the efficiency of a netball shooter by looking at the number of actions with the desired outcome divided by the total attempts, expressed as a percentage (i.e. 3 out of 4 attempts and 75% shooting accuracy). For additional examples of the most common ways to evaluate efficiency readers should see Palao and Morante (2013), where there are examples from several types of sports (e.g. invasion, batting and field and net and/or wall). Whilst establishing the data requirements of a system, analysts must also consider the types of video sequences that are needed to be viewed to support effective

DOI: 10.4324/9781003375463-5

video feedback to coaches and players. This may require an analyst to identify qualitative video sequences linked to their team's game model (principles) in addition to technical indicators.

Once the most important part of system development (i.e. discussions with coaching staff) has taken place, analysts are then able to commence system design. Within applied coaching and analysis settings, there are a significant number of commercial software packages that can be used to develop analysis systems, and these include Hudl SportsCode (Hudl, Lincoln, NE), Angles (Fulcrum Technologies, Bellevue, WA), Nacsport (Nacsport, Gran Canaria, Spain), Focus (Catapult Sports, Melbourne, Australia), Play (Metrica Sports, Amsterdam, Netherlands), Dartfish Pro (Dartfish, Fribourg, Switzerland), LongoMatch (Fluendo, Barcelona, Spain) and My Video Analyser (My Video Analyser, Hertogenbosch, Netherlands). Fundamentally, each software allows the ingest of video files and provides the analyst with the ability to observe and record data at a behavioural level. However, there are differences in the way each software package collects, processes and outputs information and video. The next part of this chapter describes and compares the functionality of three commercial analysis packages, Hudl SportsCode, Angles and Nacsport and how these can be used to develop manually operated computerised analysis systems.

Computerised system design

Readers will already be familiar with the three types of manual hand notation system: sequential systems, frequency tables and scatter diagrams described in Chapter 4. Computerised systems offer more flexibility when processing data from sequential systems into summary frequency tables, and scatter diagrams can be used to collect event locations alongside additional event data (e.g. event type, time and outcome). Nevertheless, the principles of hand notation are extremely helpful in supporting the translation of an existing (hand notation) system to a computerised system, or the development of a new computerised system from scratch. Transitioning to computerised software, the starting point for analysts in commercial software is the 'blank canvas' presented by a Code Window (Hudl SportsCode), Category Template (Nacsport) or Mark Up (Angles) and the requirement to add and configure a series of event buttons for data entry input. A recommendation is to start with pen and paper and sketch out some ideas, before jumping into a computerised software package. The following sections will cover event types used to represent behaviour, link types/button actions and specialist features (e.g. scatter diagrams and heat maps) used to represent event locations.

Data entry (input)

Within Hudl SportsCode, analysts can add a series of buttons to a Code Window and configure as code buttons or text labels. A timed code button can be set with a 5 s lead and 5 s lag time, and once pressed will record a 10 s clip that populates the timeline. This is useful when an analyst wishes to record an individual event such as a pass or tackle in soccer. A toggle code button can be used to code discrete events that have no set duration, an example of this would be a team's possession, which is commonly coded in all invasion sports. An analyst would code the event by starting and stopping the code button manually. It is possible to use a lead time of 5 s at the start of the clip, this is really with playback in mind that if the analyst were to show the clip back, it would not start abruptly. However, if manual code buttons are being used to collect time-based data to generate information such as duration of time spent in zones (e.g., pitch areas), the analyst must be aware that the use of lead and lag times will impact the values. Text labels are used to add additional information to describe code button (events), for example, if a user has a code button for a scrum or lineout set piece event in rugby union, a text label of 'won' or 'lost' may be added to denote the outcome. Multiple text labels can be added to a coded event for further detail, expanding on the previous example, this may include an area of the pitch (e.g. own 22, own 22 to halfway, halfway to opposition 22 or opposition 22) or type of lineout (e.g. five-man or seven-man).

Data entry in Angles is undertaken using a Mark Up Window with clip buttons that are configured with mark-up or mark-down times and qualifiers. Time down can be set with a positive or negative value, commonly this will be a negative value (e.g. −5 s) and when pressed it will subtract that time from the play head and start marking the clip on the timeline. Time up will add a time value (e.g. 5 s) to the end of clip. Both mark-up and mark-down can be used together to add any length of time to the start and end of clips. When using buttons in this way, the analyst will see the clip added to the timeline (n.b. it will look visually different depending on the different use of time up and time down) and will need to stop the clip themselves. The 'auto-up' option is a way to add a timed mark up to the timeline, therefore if used with a −5 s time down and a duration of 10 s, this will create a 15 s clip in total on the timeline, the difference here is the analyst does not need to close off the button.

Like text labels in Hudl SportsCode, within Angles it is possible to describe events and add additional information using qualifiers. A strength of the qualifier is that it adds a timestamp at the exact moment a button is pressed and is extremely useful when working with data exports such as comma-separated values (CSV) text files. As well as the qualifier name, an additional layer of information can be included called a 'Category'. There is a similar feature within the Code Window of Hudl SportsCode and Button Template of Nacsport, where text labels / descriptors can be attributed to a 'Group'. This additional layer of information is helpful when working with the analysis facilities and data exports.

To register events in Nacsport, an analyst must create a Button Template with a series of category and descriptor buttons. A manual mode category button allows the analyst to start and stop a button themselves, very much like manual code buttons (Hudl SportsCode) and mark up and down (Angles).

Categories can be set with pre and post times, therefore if a Category button is set with 5 s pre and 5 s post, when it is clicked, it will create a 10 s register. Descriptors add extra detail to categories and function the same as text labels (Hudl SportsCode) and Qualifiers (Angles). Nacsport descriptors are also timestamped like qualifiers in Angles and can be exported as a Microsoft Excel file (.XLS Format). Timestamped descriptors (and qualifiers from Angles) will be discussed later in this chapter.

Nacsport provides two separate functions when inputting data, the vertical play-by-play function where registers can be viewed or edited during input, or a dynamic timeline where data from a category window populates a timeline. Hudl SportsCode and Angles populate timelines directly from the Code Window and Mark Up respectively and allow viewing and editing of events on the timeline (i.e. adding, deleting or adjusting). All three software packages have the capability to allow real-time data entry whilst a video is being recorded (live) or via a short time delay. For example, an analyst can enter data 30 s behind live play, with access to full video control capabilities to pause, rewind and then catch up with play. Analysis systems developed for use in real-time may focus on the collection of critical match events, with post-event team and individual systems used to collect further information.

Overall, there are similarities in the way events at a team or individual level are recorded and described in each software package. The main differences are the timestamp of events and sub-groupings that can be included to add further layers of information. Furthermore, there are features within each software such as link types, button actions and ways to enter event locations (e.g. scatter diagrams) that can support ergonomic data entry. These will be discussed in the next section.

Link types & button actions

The following section will describe the use of various link types (Hudl SportsCode and Nacsport) and button actions (Angles) and their role in data system design and data entry. Data entry in Hudl SportsCode can be expedited using activation and exclusive links. Similarly, this can be achieved in Nacsport using a series of activation links and exclusions. Events can be exclusively linked together when we know only one event can occur at a given time. Using soccer possession as an example, only one team can have possession of the ball at a time, two manual event buttons named 'Team A Possession' and 'Team B Possession' can be exclusively linked meaning when one is active the other is deactivated. Similarly, using the down up and up down button actions in Angles, it is possible to toggle between buttons (e.g. Team A Possession and Team B Possession) when pressed down or up to achieve the same outcome of only having one active event.

During the possession, other events such as final third entries, crosses and attempts on goal can occur. Activation links can be used to record these events alongside the broader possession clip. For example, if 'Team A Possession' is active and a shot on goal occurs, a text label (SportsCode) or descriptor (Nacsport) can describe the outcome (e.g. on target, off target, blocked or goal). An activation link can be added from 'on target' to a timed (10 s lead and 5 s lag time) event button called Team A Shot. A longer lead time is used in this example, with the end video clip in mind and a desire to see the build in the lead up to the shot. When the descriptor 'on target' is pressed, it will activate 'Team A Shot', creating the event and adding the descriptor to both open events. A similar chain of notation can be used in Angles with an auto-up button for 'Team A Shot' (including a −10 s time down and 5 s duration) and a down action from the qualifier 'on target' to the button 'Team A Shot'. 'On target' will trigger the 'Team A Shot' button and the qualifier 'on target' will be added to this button and 'Team A Possession'.

Extending the description above, Figure 5.1 shows a simple SportsCode soccer possession template using a series of exclusive links, activation link types and six additional code buttons for possession in pitch zones (e.g., Def, Mid & Att). In this example, the analyst would only be required to click on one of the six buttons at a time to collect possession-based data. At any one point, only two buttons will be active (one pitch zone and one team possession button), to end both events at the same time, the analyst would press the tab key on their keyboard. A combination of code buttons and link types are useful as a basis to team-based analysis templates for invasion sports (e.g. soccer, rugby union and field hockey) where possession in zones is important to record. To further develop the example, additional events and text labels could be added. Readers should note it is also possible to develop the same system presented in Figure 5.1 within both Nacsport and Angles.

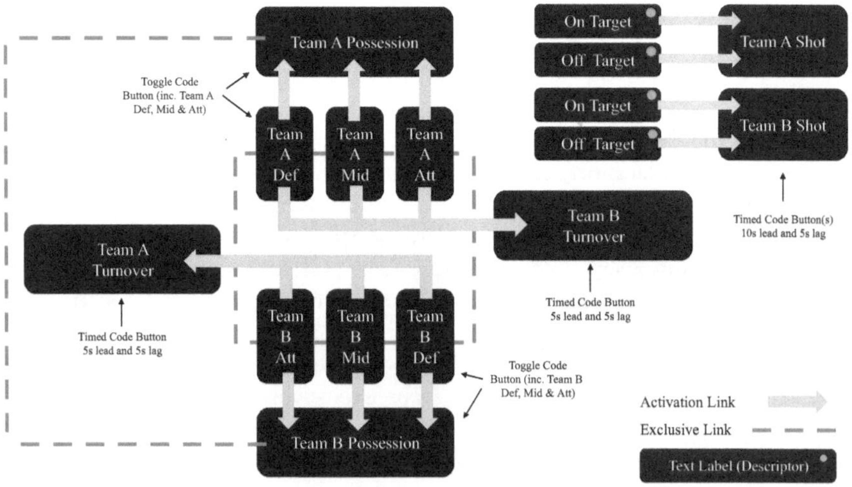

Figure 5.1 Basic principles of a soccer possession template in Hudl SportsCode.

In all three software packages, active events (i.e. code, category and clip buttons) can receive either a single text label, descriptor or qualifier or multiple. Also, each software package has the capability to block information from event buttons where required. This is helpful when trying to manage the distribution of data being collected by an analysis system. Nacsport buttons can also be 'clustered' which involves layering Category and Descriptor buttons on top of one another and when the button at the top is clicked it will act as an activation chain to the buttons beneath. The order of the buttons is controlled using the 'vertical lock' settings within the button properties with the highest number, e.g. 'five', representing the top button and the lowest number, e.g., 'one', being the bottom.

By successfully implementing link types and button actions, data collection can be expedited, the transfer of data into events can be controlled and the number of 'clicks' required to input data can be reduced. As well as link types and button actions, there are also additional features that aid data entry and user navigation of analysis systems, these will be described in the next section.

Graphical User Interface (GUI): navigation features

In Nacsport, buttons can be added to a series of panels and once buttons are clicked the system will navigate to a different panel (creating a chain between panels) to support data entry. Angles has a slightly different way to achieve this, but the principle is very similar. Down and Up Centre Button Actions assist users navigate (swipe) to different areas of the template. The advantages of these subtle features within each package are as follows: (1) it reduces the need to have a large template filling the computer screen, and (2) it creates a 'chain of notation' regarding the input of data. Using Nacsports panels feature as an example, this could be player (Number 8) > event (Pass) > pitch location (Mid Zone) > outcome (Successful). The home panel would have a series of timed player category buttons and then a subsequent panel for event action, pitch location and outcome, all of which would be descriptors. As the analyst inputs information, a new panel is triggered, once the final piece of information is added (e.g. outcome), the analyst is automatically returned to the home panel to commence data entry for another player. This systematic data entry process maintains the order and structure of data, which is helpful when the exact sequence and time of events are required. In addition, this approach can also reduce data input errors and improve reliability. To contextualise, Figure 5.2 displays how information would appear within the video clip on the timeline of each software and the data (table) structures, including timestamp of qualifiers (Angles) and descriptors (Nacsport).

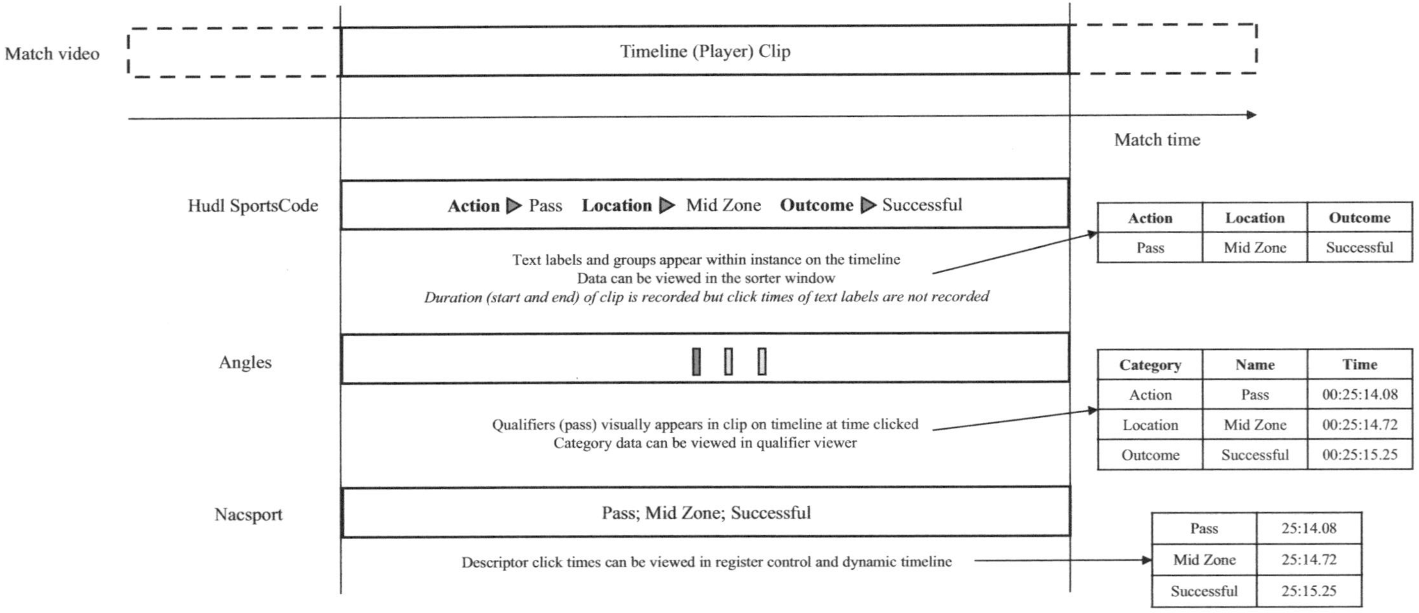

Figure 5.2 Input of event data in Hudl SportsCode, Angles and Nacsport.

In summary, the data entry features described to this point all contribute to the successful collection of time-based data (e.g. possession areas), and frequency and outcome of events (e.g. number of passes, number of completed passes or shots on and off target). This type of information is widely used by coaches to measure team and individual performances and support the identification of video feedback. However, desire for more granular level information on player and team events has led to the development of features within commercial video analysis packages that allow the collection of event location data. The next section will discuss the processes and software features that enable this form of data collection.

Event location data

Although the individual player analysis example in the previous section provided a good level of information, when recording events (e.g. pass, shots, tackles, interceptions and dribbles), a more detailed and ordered sequence of player actions can be recorded. Therefore, as well as the event type, events can be described by the time and location (X and Y coordinates) where the action took place on the playing pitch (Klemp, 2021). Depending on the type of the event, information such as the start and end location for a pass or the outcome of a tackle can be recorded.

The Cartesian (Angles), Graphic Descriptor (Nacsport) and Heat Map Graph Type (Hudl SportsCode) are powerful features that can be integrated into Mark Up Windows, Category Templates and Code Windows to collect x and y data. To operationalise this in Angles, a Cartesian pitch button must be set as an 'attribute' in the Mark-Up Window. Attributes allow additional information to be collected on events, with the additional data appearing as a separate column of data in the attribute editor. Using soccer and the FIFA recommend pitch size dimensions of 105m (length) and 68m (width) as an example, a soccer pitch can be set with the Cartesian scale of 105 (x axis) and 68 (y axis) and a step value of one. The step value goes up in a value of 1 m each time and acts as a grid reference overlaid over the pitch. Each time an event is mapped to the pitch it will return an x and y value (e.g. 45, 19), conceptually shown in Figure 5.3. In comparison, the process to set up and use a Graphic Descriptor (Nacsport) and Heat Map (Hudl SportsCode) to collect x and y co-ordinates is similar. An added benefit of collecting x and y data in Nacsport and Hudl SportsCode is that each software can (1) visualise events as heat maps, and (2) allow individual events (videos) to be viewed directly from the heat map visualisation. This type of interactivity between data and video can help support the identification of video clips for feedback purposes. Furthermore, all three packages have the ability to export x and y data for use in specialist data visualisation programs such as Tableau or Power Bi.

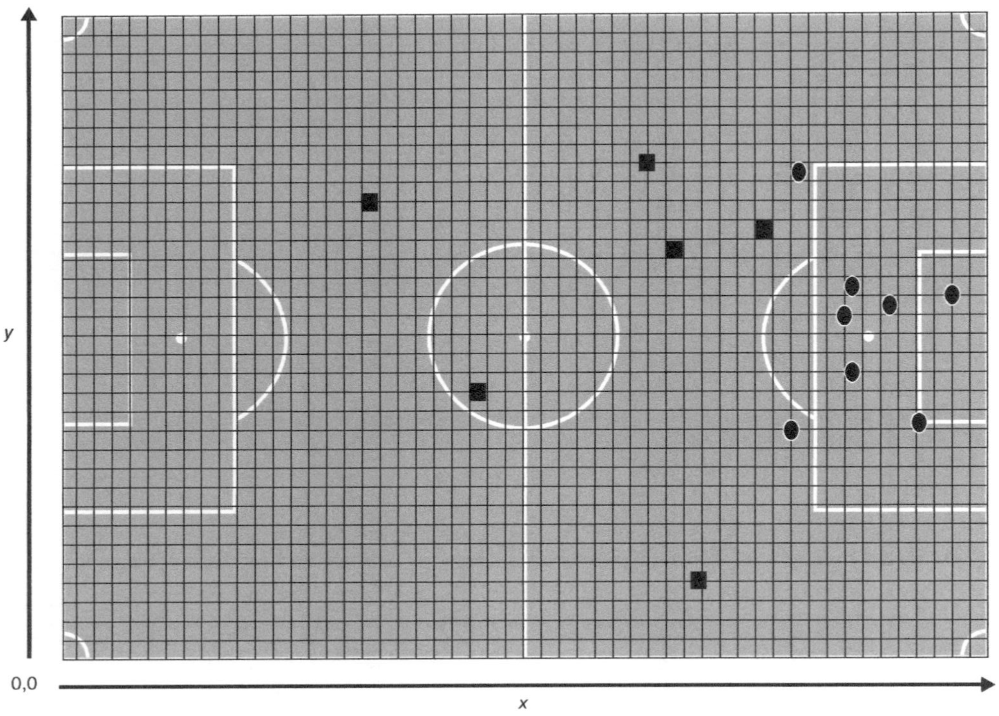

Player	Event	X	Y
A	Shot	91	46
A	Shot	88	44
B	Shot	83	64
A	Shot	87	56
A	Shot	97	43
B	Shot	83	24
A	Shot	95	65
A	Shot	87	39
B	Pass	60	22
B	Pass	67	39
A	Pass	80	31
A	Pass	67	87
B	Pass	30	31
A	Pass	44	55

■ Pass ● Shot

Figure 5.3 x and y coordinates for ball event data in soccer.

Some readers will already have some knowledge of x and y event level data, prior to reading this chapter, whereas others may be more unfamiliar with the concept. Readers or analysts with a particular interest in soccer will likely be aware of advanced metrics such as expected goals (xG) and expected assists (xA). Expected goals (xG), the quality of chances in soccer has received significant attention due to the fact some shots are deemed better than others and are more likely to result in a goal. To develop probability models, each shot is assigned an x and y value. However, shots on goal in soccer are infrequent compared to other actions in the game. Therefore, interest has led to the annotation of other on the ball events, such as passing (Van Haaren, 2019). For this reason x and y coordinates can be used to record detailed soccer passing data, this could either be a whole passing sequence of a team or all the passes including origin, end point and outcome of an individual player. The ability of Angles and Nacsport to record the exact time of an event (using a qualifier / descriptor) does differentiate both packages from Hudl SportsCode, where it is only possible to record the location of event or describe an event with a text label (e.g. Pass > Successful). Refer to Figure 5.2 for a representation of the data table structures in each software. Subsequently, having the exact timestamp of an event is extremely powerful and can aid the calculation and extraction of time-based performance indicators. Using soccer, the following example describes a way to analyse a team's ability to regain the ball after losing possession.

Regaining the ball in soccer (transition)

Teams who are deemed high pressing strive to regain the ball in less than 6 s, an approach popularised by Pep Guardiola when he was the manager of FC Barcelona 2008–12. Conceptually, this coaching idea can be taken and turned it into a performance indicator. A common way to do this in commercial software (without time stamped event data) is splitting the pitch up into a series of broad zones to record the number of times a team regains the ball in each zone after losing possession (Barreira, 2014; Cooper and Pulling, 2020). The data can be visually presented to support the evaluation of a team's 'pressing' capabilities and identify video clips to be shown in pre- or post-match briefings. To 'quantify' the metric differently, a code or category event (e.g. Def Transition) containing a series of descriptors (Nacsport) or qualifiers/attributes (Angles) can be used to record the time and location of the event (x, y). Using a timestamp for 'ball lost' and 'ball regained', it would be possible to visually record the event and extract time-based data to calculate time differences between qualifiers/descriptors. In the case of Nacsport, it is also possible to use the descriptor calculate (within the timeline) to return the frequency as a 'new descriptor' back into the Matrix (a which feature which will be discussed in more detail in the next section). Therefore, if a team had 50 ball recoveries in match, regain time (30 in under 6 s and 20 requiring 6.01 s or longer), now defined by descriptors (e.g. ball recovery <6 & ball recovery greater than 6) would appear in matrix, making it easy to access the video clips for review.

This is a short post-hoc process that needs to be completed after registering all events from a given match. Alternatively, the data can be exported out of both packages to allow the calculation of descriptive statistics; minimum, maximum, range and central tendencies such mean, mode or median in specialist programs such as Microsoft Excel. In summary, if a coach requires information on ball recoveries that take less than 6 s, there are strategies to achieve this. Analysts should consider if data alone are enough, or if video is needed? Ultimately, to comprehensively evaluate a team's pressing ability the exact spatial movements of all players and the ball are needed, which is only available from camera tracking systems. Nonetheless, being able to collect ball event data with event type, timestamp and spatial location in commercial software provides great opportunities for analysts.

Though the section has used soccer as an illustrative example, it is possible to collect detailed event data in other invasion sports as well as individual sports. Despite the potential to enhance data collection, the process is not without error and can be time consuming, therefore analysts should consider if the benefits outweigh the time commitments required to implement the data collection.

Data entry (input): summary

In summary, all the features have an important role to play in the development of effective and efficient data collection systems. However, it is important these facilitate the analysis system to meet the information needs of the coaching process but also collect a rich layer of meta-data to support the analysis of performance. To consolidate knowledge and understanding of the features and terminology within this section, they have been summarised in Table 5.1. Moving forward, the next section will consider the analysis facilities available to support data processing and interactive video feedback.

Table 5.1 Summary of data input features and terminology

Software Feature	*Hudl SportsCode*	*Angles*	*Nacsport*
Data Input	*Code Template*	*Mark Up Window*	*Category Template*
Types of buttons available to record and describe events.	**Code buttons** add events (instances) to the timeline **Text labels** add additional information to events.	**Clip buttons** mark events in the timeline **Qualifiers** describe additional actions that happen within a clip. **Attributes** add additional detail to qualifiers. An example of this Cartesian feature set.	**Category buttons** register events in the register control and timeline **Descriptor buttons** add additional information to categories

(*Continued*)

Table 5.1 (Continued)

Software Feature	*Hudl SportsCode*	*Angles*	*Nacsport*
Data Input	*Code Template*	*Mark Up Window*	*Category Template*
Link types and actions for navigation	Activation, Deactivation and Exclusive Links	Actions (Down > Up, Centre, Centre & Down, Up and Up, Down & Down and Private Action)	Activation, Deactivation and Exclusions Cluster & Panel Flows
x and y (co-ordinate) event data entry	Heat Map (chart type)	Cartesian Feature (attribute)	Graphic Descriptor

Throughput: analysis facilities

Once a system has been used to analyse performance, a series of analysis facilities support the processing of data and interactive video feedback. The following section will describe the function of the Matrix in each software, and specialist features such as the Sorter Window (Hudl SportsCode), Data Table (Angles) and Play-by-Play Table (Nacsport).

Matrix

A Matrix allows the cross tabulation of coded timeline events with text labels (Hudl SportsCode) and descriptors (Nacsport), and is one of the most common analysis facilities in commercial packages. A strength of the matrix tool in Hudl SportsCode and Nacsport is the ability to use Boolean Operators (AND, OR, NOT) to combine or exclude variables when creating new columns of data. This provides interactivity between data and video, making it extremely easy to review video clips and add clips to a video presentation (video presentations are discussed in more detail later in this chapter). Unfortunately, the functionality to combine qualifiers is not available within the Angles Matrix, thus reducing the scope of its use. Furthermore, Nacsport (Clip Filter) and Angles (Filters) are features that allow events to be searched on the timeline and added to video presentations.

Figure 5.4 displays a Matrix with event data for a basketball player and the Boolean Operators that have been used to organise the data. In reference to the shooting statistics 2-point, 3-point and free throw, a descriptor called 'Missed' has been used to describe unsuccessful shots, otherwise the shot attempt was successful. By clicking on any of the events, it would be possible to watch the clips back. Matrix data can also be exported into programs such Microsoft Excel to calculate performance indicator values such as shooting percentages for 2-point (15/20 = 75%), 3-point (6/8 = 75%) and Free Throw (4/7 = 57%). Spreadsheet packages also provide options to visualise data in charts and tables. A common analysis workflow includes exporting the Matrix Data into a raw 'data dump' sheet in Excel, which automatically

	MATRIX																
	2 Point OR 3 Point OR Free Throw	Missed	2 Point NOT Missed	2 Point AND Missed	2 Point	3 Point NOT Missed	3 Point AND Missed	3 Point	Free Throw NOT Missed	Free Throw AND Missed	Free Throw	Offensive Rebound	Defensive Rebound	Assist	Personal Foul	Turnover	Steals
Player 1	35	10	15	5	20	6	2	8	4	3	7	4	5	2	1	3	2

Figure 5.4 Matrix data for basketball player.

processes the data and creates an output report or dashboard, a process that should take no longer than a few minutes to complete. The process is made even easier by the fact any modified matrix in Hudl SportsCode or Nacsport can be saved so it can be used match-to-match.

Event and data tables

Event and data tables display a chronologically ordered list of events from the timeline. An example of throughput interactivity is the Sorter Window in Hudl SportsCode, which can be populated with all clips from a timeline or selected rows. Within the Sorter Window, labels are listed in columns, either 'ungrouped' or under the 'group' assigned to the button during the development of the Code Window. The 'group' name is very helpful when exporting data to Microsoft Excel, as maintaining the order of the clips allows the use of pivot tables without any data processing. Similarly, Angles includes a Data Table that displays columns of data for qualifiers, categories (if used) and attribute data. Again, when exported to Microsoft Excel, these data can be processed using pivot tables. Readers will be familiar with the strengths of pivot tables and the ability to transform qualitative data into quantitative data from Chapter 4. Chronologically ordered events in Nacsport can be viewed in the play-by-play table in the registering environment. Although descriptors are listed within one clip register, rather than grouped like the Sorter Window (Hudl SportsCode) or Data Table (Angles), it is still possible to view descriptor groups in the matrix, and export event data chronologically via the timeline. A point of note is that the organisation of input data in columns (groups) is facilitated during the design of a Code Window (Hudl SportsCode), Mark Up (Angles) or Category Template (Nacsport). Additional benefits of organising data within the software are that it reduces the volume of processing needed once files are exported into Microsoft Excel. Even without using the features discussed, all three software packages have various exports that can be used to extract the chronological order of events for further data processing and visualisation. Any event lists exported from the three packages will also include the x and y event location data should this be required.

Throughput: analysis facilities (summary)

In summary, the current section has outlined various types of analysis features and exports that exist within the three software packages. These analysis features aid the identification of video clips for presentations and provide flexible data exports to support additional data processing tasks such as reports and dashboards. Whilst it is advantageous to extract data from each software packages, each software has various in-built presentation output features that can be used to visually present data and video. Table 5.2 summarises the features.

Outputs: data & video

As demonstrated in the previous section, a fundamental function of general-purpose commercial analysis packages is the interactivity between data and video feedback. The following section outlines the features available within Hudl SportsCode, Angles and Nacsport to visually present data and create edited presentations.

Table 5.2 Summary of throughputs and analysis facilities

Software Feature	*Hudl SportsCode*	*Angles*	*Nacsport*
Ability to cross tab events with descriptions for video playback.	**Matrix and matrix organiser** with ability to combine variables. Matrix data can be exported as.csv file	**Basic matrix** but no ability to combine qualifiers. Matrix data can be exported as.csv file **Filters** – search clip qualifiers and attributes within the timeline	**Matrix**, sub matrix and descriptor combinations to combine descriptors. Matrix data can be exported as.xls file **Clip filter** – search clips using descriptor combinations to combine descriptors
Chronological order of events with access to video and data	**Sorter window** displays clips in chronological order with text labels in columns. Sorter window and/ or full Edit List of timeline events can be exported as .csv file	**Data table** which includes category and attribute data (but no video link) Data table can be exported as.csv	**Play-by-play** table displays clips in chronological order with ability to edit, search and delete data. Chronological list of timeline events can be exported as .xls file.

Interactive video feedback and visualisation

Examples of interactive data and video presentation is the report mode (output) window in Hudl Sportscode and Nacsport's Dashboard feature. Common functions to display data include chart types (e.g. bar, stacked bar and pie chart) and the ability to display numerical outputs, combine variables (e.g. text labels in Hudl SportsCode and descriptors in Nacsport) and use mathematical calculations to generate percentage values. Output windows and dashboards can be split to look at data from various periods of matches (e.g., first, second, third or fourth quarter in basketball) and can be used post-event or live. Post-event data can be displayed for either one single match or multiple matches. A popular visualisation is the use of RAG – or red, amber, green statuses that function as traffic light alerts to draw attention to key performance indicator values. Typically, red signifies an area that may need attention, amber implies caution and green would suggest everything is as expected. It is important that these values are well considered; therefore, it may be beneficial to look at Butterworth's book (2023c), where he outlines a method to evaluate single match data based on typical match performance. If used in a live setting, coaches and analysts must identify what information is needed to support decision making, which may be less than that required in a post-match analysis.

The major difference between the two software packages is that Hudl SportsCode requires the analyst to have knowledge and understanding of the program's scripting language. In contrast, Nacsport negates the need to learn a coding language, therefore developing a Dashboard output for use can be expedited. Both report output windows (with scripting) and dashboards are extremely powerful and allow analysts to tailor the analysis process and presentation to their specific needs. They can greatly enhance the efficiency and effectiveness of the analysis workflow by automating repetitive tasks and providing dynamic and interactive outputs for players and coaches.

In summary, it is important to consider points raised earlier in this chapter on knowing the purpose of the system and the required information and video outputs. Readers with an interest in the functionality available within Scripting should see Chapter 5 'Statistical Windows' by O'Donoghue and Holmes (2015: 85–115) for further assistance. In addition, readers should access the support files provided by both Hudl SportsCode and Nacsport to help the implementation of these features into their own analysis systems. Angles does not currently include an interactive data or video dashboard; however, with the software's capabilities to collect rich sets of data, it may not be long before a similar feature is added to the software. Table 5.3 compares the packages with respect to these features.

Table 5.3 Interactive data visualisation and video playback

Software Feature	*Hudl SportsCode*	*Angles*	*Nacsport*
Interactive data visualisation and video playback	Using a specialised scripting language, it is possible to include scripts within buttons in the Code Window to return, calculate and display information in numerical and graphical format based on information in the timeline.	n/a	Built from the interface of the software, dashboards can display data in the form of labels, charts and graphs based on the data in the dynamic timeline.

Edited video sequences and presentations

There are several types of edited video types that can be created by analysts (O'Donoghue, 2006), and some common examples include the preview of an upcoming opposition or a post-match review. Table 5.4 provides an overview of the video presentation features available within various software packages. These features allow analysts to create and deliver edited video highlights without having to leave the software package. Remaining within the software package for playback is particularly advantageous when working with multiple video angles as it is possible to seamlessly switch between angles (e.g. wide, TV/tight or behind goal angles) during playback. Presenting from within the software also affords coaches and analysts the opportunity to use the native video controls of the software.

Table 5.4 Video presentation features

Software Feature	*Hudl SportsCode*	*Angles*	*Nacsport*
Create edited video presentations within software package	Movie Organiser and Sorter Window	Composer	Presentations
Video annotations and/or telestration	Hudl Studio is an integrated telestration tool that allows users to quickly add professional, dynamic drawings and graphics to video angles.	n/a	Klipdraw Motion is an integrated telestration tool that can be used in presentations to highlight key moments and add drawings, animations and tracked graphics.

Video clips can be moved directly from timelines and matrices into the Movie Organiser (Hudl SportsCode), Composer (Angles) and Presentations (Nacsport). Once added, all packages allow clips to be reorganised into different themes and sub-themes and edited (e.g. length of time). Using soccer as an example, an analysis presentation may be built around a team's game model (i.e. principles of play) and include video clips on tactical team-based situations when 'in possession', 'out of possession' and 'in transition' (from attack to defence and defence to attack). Defending and attacking set pieces (e.g. corners and free kicks) are of great analytical interest to coaches and players. Individual player clips can also be added, and these could be split into strengths and areas to exploit if looking at opposition players, or strengths and areas for development if reviewing a player on your own team.

Standard annotation tools (e.g. lines, arrows and circles) are available within SportsCode, Nacsport and Angles. However, SportsCode (Studio) and Nacsport (Klipdraw) respectively have enhanced telestration drawing tools integrated into their software that can be used to add visually engaging graphics over video. Angles does not have integrated video telestration; however, analysts are able to add simple annotation using Preview, a built-in image and PDF viewer on macOS. Extending on this, analysts can also use Adobe Photoshop or Adobe Infinity; however, these programs do not facilitate 'video telestration'. Principles and use of specialist video telestration packages are discussed in more depth in Chapter 7 of this book, and readers should peruse this for further information and applied examples.

Title slides can be added within a presentation to provide structure when moving to and from different sections of presentation. A popular function is the use of 'notes', which allows coaches and analysts to add short text descriptions to a video clip, these act as a prompt during live presentations or when viewing clips or the whole presentation outside of the software. A popular workflow available within all three packages is the ability to import presentation slides from other presentation programs (e.g. Microsoft PowerPoint or iWork Keynote). These packages along with programs such as Adobe Photoshop and InDesign can be used to create visually appealing presentation slides, a common visualisation to create and import are formation graphics with player shirts or headshots. There may be a requirement to include data visualisation in the form of charts and tables; again, these can be created in specialist programs such as Microsoft Excel, Power Bi or Tableau and imported. A downside of this is the loss of interactivity; if this is important, analysts can use the interactive features of Report Windows with scripting (SportsCode), dashboards (Nacsport) discussed in the previous section as part of presentation and feedback sessions.

Standalone videos (e.g. edited sequences or playlists) can be exported to be played in media players or other presentation programs (e.g. Microsoft PowerPoint or iWork Keynote) external of the software packages. There are additional post-hoc processes (e.g. video conversion) and time required to facilitate these which analysts should be aware of. It is also common to share full match or edited videos to online sharing platforms that are accessible on smart devices (e.g. Hudl Online, Nacsport Hub or Coach Logic). Uploading to an online platform requires the video and associated XML file, the process is seamless if there is a sufficient internet connection to facilitate the process.

Outputs: video and data (summary)

In summary, there are a variety of integrated data and video presentation features within each software package. Regardless of capabilities, the presentation and feedback requirements will differ for all individuals (e.g. analysts, coaches and players), hence there is no universal approach stronger than another. Therefore, analysts should consider which features are the most suitable for helping coaches and players make decisions on different aspects of performance, and the communication of feedback.

Even though this chapter has successfully outlined the data entry input, analysis facilities and output capabilities of Hudl SportsCode, Angles and Nacsport, there are considerations that analysts need to be aware of prior to data collection and the use of video analysis with coaches and players. The final section of this chapter will now cover the importance of system testing and approaches to ensuring accuracy of data collection.

System testing and consistency checking

The cornerstone of any computerised performance analysis systems is reliable and accurate data collection. This is because the information collected by the system is used to inform decisions about pre-match, in-game and post-match player performance and feedback. Throughout system development, analysts should engage in pilot testing to help resolve any issues that may arise before the system is used in a coaching setting. It would be beneficial to involve the coach in this process, and this will ensure the system is delivering the required information and video. Once completed, analysts will then be ready to use the system to collect, process and analyse data.

O'Donoghue and Longville (2004) drew attention to the importance of reliability in the delivery of performance analysis support and suggested 'consistency checking' should be used to improve reliability. The principle of consistency checking involves the analyst identifying and correcting data entry errors before processing performance indicators and selecting video clips to feedback to coaches and players. Examples of errors that could occur include recording an event incorrectly, missing the outcome of an event and/or attributing an event to the wrong player. Analysts should not see this as manipulation of the data, but view 'consistency checking' as part of the data input stage (O'Donoghue and Mayes, 2013).

Should analysts wish to test the reliability of an analysis system this can be achieved using various exports discussed in this chapter, and percentage error or the kappa statistics, which are recognised reliability measures in sport performance analysis (O'Donoghue, 2015: 185–192). However, due to the nature of data entry, the exports may need to be converted into a suitable format for processing a reliability assessment, particularly the kappa statistic. In cases where an analysis system is being used by multiple analysts, it is recommended that a formal reliability test be employed during the training phase to evaluate the accuracy of data collection. However, when working on a match-to-match basis, analysts are encouraged to apply 'consistency checking'. Further information on how to conduct percentage error and kappa assessments when using computerised systems can be found in O'Donoghue and Holmes (2015: 225–247).

Conclusions

This chapter has provided an overview of computerised performance analysis systems. Firstly, it discussed the types of data entry methods in various software packages (Hudl SportsCode, Angles, and Nacsport), including the different types of buttons, labels and qualifiers to represent events and add additional information. Following this, a comprehensive overview of the analysis facilities, specifically focusing on the matrix, event and data tables and how these are used were provided. This included drawing attention to various data export options. The section also covered a wide range of aspects related to presenting data and video outputs within the context of commercial video analysis software. Importantly, the section highlights the need for a systematic approach to data collection, and considerations for accuracy and reliability in performance analysis systems. Overall, the section provides insights into the capabilities and workflows of three commercial video analysis software packages and how analysts can use these to develop systems to support the delivery of video and data feedback.

6 Analysing performances using computerised systems

Introduction

This chapter describes the operation of systems once they have been developed. Three examples are discussed: the first is a system used in netball coaching, the second is a system used in academic research about soccer possessions, and the third is used to analyse decision making. It is necessary to briefly touch on the development of these systems simply because the operating environment for the systems needed to be considered during system design. The netball analysis system is operated live during matches with some supplementary data entry occurring after matches. The second system is used during post-match video analysis to record possession starts, passes and attempts on goal. The third system was also used in a research study. More importantly, this system was used to evaluate the decision making of players during Australian Rules football matches and the impact of a decision-making intervention that was being done by the squad.

Example 1. The netball analysis system

Background and development

The netball analysis system is used as an example of practical coaching because one of the authors (Peter O'Donoghue) used the system with eight different squads from 2003 to 2013. The system was originally developed in Focus X2 (Elite Sports Analysis, Dalgety Bay, UK) for use with the Welsh senior netball squad (O'Donoghue and Longville, 2004) and was also used by Welsh under 21 and under 19 squads as well as the Celtic Dragons. When O'Donoghue moved from the Celtic Dragons to Team Bath, it was necessary to implement the system in Sportscode (Hudl, Lincoln, NE) because the squad were using Apple MacIntosh computers. The system is used to record possession events, shots, scores and offensive rebounds. There are six types of possession which are characterised by how they start:

- Centre pass: this is how games start and how they restart after scores.
- Interception: where a player receives a ball played by the opponent that was intended to be received by one of the opponent's team-mates.

DOI: 10.4324/9781003375463-6

- Sideline: where the ball has gone out of play and so a team gets the equivalent of a throw-in in soccer.
- Backline: where the ball has gone out of play and so the game restarts with a free pass from behind the team's own backline.
- Defensive rebound: where an opponent has missed a shot and a defender takes the ball as it rebounds from the rim of the goal.
- Free: this is used for a variety of free throws given for footwork errors, holding the ball too long, illegal passes, obstruction and contact. This is also used on occasions where there is a toss-up that results in the team previously in possession of the ball no longer being in possession of the ball.

These possession types are exclusively linked, meaning that a new possession starting turns off the previous possession that was being recorded. Descriptor buttons are used to record the quarter each possession occurs in. When the system was implemented in Focus X2, this was applied using a "sticky button" as the events were entered. Now that the system is implemented in Sportscode, all of the events within a quarter are selected at the end of the quarter and labelled together. Goals, shots and offensive rebounds are recorded using code buttons. The code buttons for goals and shots have activation links ensuring that a descriptor is added to the current possession noting these outcomes.

Operating environments

The system has been used in different operating environments. Venue, filming location and how much time there is to turn feedback round to the coach and players all impact on data entry and analysis. The match could be filmed from a side-on view or from behind the court. Video footage from behind the court is preferable for the coaches but requires the camera operator to zoom in and out as the play moves up and down the court. This requires a separate camera operator to the analyst if the match is to be coded live. Where the match is being recorded from a side-on view, it is possible for a skilled analyst to operate the camera and code the match live. Typically, the camera does not need to zoom into the action and simply needs to swing from left to right as the play moves from left to right. The analyst can control the camera with the non-dominant hand and code the match with the dominant hand. Ergonomics is very important here; a table for the computer and a good tripod is needed. It is essential to use hot keys on the keyboard in order to code a match live while operating the camera. Viewing the match and operating the keyboard is much easier than viewing the match, using a mouse and checking the computer screen to make sure the pointer is at the right on-screen button. Each combination of team and event has a different key assigned, meaning that only one key needs to be hit when an event occurs rather than two. The choice was necessary to decide on which keys to use for different events. C and G for centre pass and goal, respectively, were natural choices, except this was only for the centre passes and goals for the team. The V and H keys were used for opponent's centre passes and goals, respectively. The reason for this is because V and H are located next to C and G on the keyboard. This was not possible for all event types. For example, I was used for team interceptions but O could not be used for opposition interceptions because it was already assigned to another event type (a sideline ball after the ball had been played out). Instead, N was used to represent opposition interceptions because it was the second letter of "interception". We'll not go through the rest of the keys assigned to different events. It sounds complicated but when using the system over a season, the analyst gets used to the keys. Indeed, when events were being performed during matches, the analyst was mentally thinking of them in terms of letters. There are occasions where the analyst might make a mistake during coding. It is not possible to correct this live as subsequent events need to be coded. Therefore, the system uses the space bar to record where the operator believes an error has occurred. This allows the analyst to quickly locate any errors and correct them after match quarters or after the match.

After the match, the coding can be checked to ensure that the events follow the syntax rules for the sport. The centre passes need to alternate between the two teams. Turnovers between centre passes need to alternate. A shot, goal or offensive rebound can only occur within a possession for the team performing the event. Any errors with respect to these syntax rules can easily be detected through filtering events, allowing them to be corrected in the 15–20 minutes after the match. During this period, the players will be doing their cool down and changing. It is particularly busy where the analyst may appear to be antisocial, but the fact is that a complete correctly coded video of the match needs to be ready to copy onto the coaches' computers before everyone leaves the venue.

There are some venues where it is not possible for the equipment used to be connected to a mains power supply. Usually, the batteries for the camera and computer being used last for an entire netball match. However, there can be problems if there are additional tasks being done by the computer that require more CPU (central processing unit) usage and hence more power. For example, an additional screen might be attached to the computer so that delayed video can be displayed. Copying video frames and sending them to an additional screen will use additional power and could result in the computer running out of battery before the match has completed. In such a situation, the analyst will need to get to a mains power supply soon after the match, code the remaining video recorded by the camera and join the two coded videos together. This might not be straightforward and can delay time to feedback.

The squad may need to consider the relative value of using an extra screen for a delayed video display during the match against having information for feedback sooner rather than later.

While working as Team Bath analyst, O'Donoghue also used the system with the England under 21 and senior squads until 2013. At this point, Andrew Butterworth was appointed as the England squad's analyst and the system was extended considerably to take advantage of the latest technologies (Butterworth, 2023a, 2023c). A statistical window was coded to determine percentage conversion rates for each type of possession live during the match. These conversion rates were presented in an output viewer window that was sent wirelessly to a device being used by a coach on the bench. The statistical window in Sportscode uses underlying programme code created by the analyst to examine the timeline and produce higher order statistics. It can also be used to add descriptors to the timeline without the user needing to code them. O'Donoghue and Holmes (2015: 85–115) show how this can be used to automatically update the score in tennis. Additional events of interest to netball coaches were coded live by a second analyst or coach using an iPad device. The iPad communicated with the main analyst's computer during the match so that these additional events could be included in the match timeline. Ball touches by individual players were coded in the 24 hours after the match. This was a highly skilled process that required familiarity with the players within the squad and the opposing squads. Once coded, these touches could be checked relatively quickly for a player at a time. Displaying video sequences for the touches coded for an individual player makes it reasonably obvious if there is a touch that has been coded for the player where, in fact, another player performed the touch. The wealth of information recorded allowed multimedia profiles to be produced for the players. These profiles interactively presented quantitative information about performances as well as video sequences (Butterworth, 2023c).

Reliability

Reliability is arguably more important in practical performance analysis than it is in scientific research. This is because the analysis will be used to inform decisions made by coaches and players about preparation for important matches. The reliability of the system includes the whole process of operating the system, including correcting errors at the end of the match. The error checking and correcting steps should not be seen as a way of covering up limited reliability. These steps are part of the process that leads to the information that the coaches and players will use.

Analysis and feedback

The code buttons were for team and possession type pairs and these are used as the rows of a matrix produced for each match coded in the system.

Match quarters and event outcomes are clustered to form the columns of the matrix. The matrix is exported from the video analysis software and the frequencies pasted into a pre-programmed spreadsheet to determine percentage conversion rates as shown in Figure 6.1. Figure 6.1 is a summary sheet that is given to the coaches about 30 minutes after the match. This has merged interceptions and defensive rebounds into a single possession class called "Live turnovers". The frees, sidelines and backlines are merged into a second broad possession class of turnover called "Restart turnovers". The difference between a restart turnover and a live turnover is that there is a stoppage in play before a restart possession commences. This allows both teams to set their players up in preparation for the possession. A live turnover, on the other hand, is where a team takes the ball from the opponent and play continues without any stoppage being signalled by the umpires. The statistics for the team's own possessions reflect their attacking play and higher values are desired rather than lower values. The statistics for the opposition's possessions reflect the team's defensive performance and lower values are preferable. The example in Figure 6.1 shows where the coach circles particular possession types to represent good play. The rectangles are drawn where the coach identifies areas where improvement is needed. The coach can mark the sheet in less than a minute based on the statistics but also on having watched the match from the bench. The marked statistics give the analyst direction on which video sequences to include within highlights videos. You will see that nothing is marked on the overall turnover rows; this is because these statistics are made up from the live and restart turnovers. Considering the team's own possessions, you will see that the coach marked restart turnovers in the fourth quarter where the conversion rate was 67% but did not make live turnovers in the first and fourth quarters even though they also had a conversion rate of 67%. The issue here

Match: Date:					
Team	Match	Q1	Q2	Q3	Q4
Centre Passes to Goal	32/51=63%	8/13=62%	7/12=58%	11/14=79%	6/12=50%
Restart T/Overs to Goal	12/23=52%	4/7=57%	3/5=60%	1/5=20%	4/6=67%
Live T/Overs to Goal	10/16=63%	2/3=67%	2/5=40%	4/5=80%	2/3=67%
All T/Overs to Goal	22/39=56%	6/10=60%	5/10=50%	5/10=50%	6/9=67%
Opposition	Match	Q1	Q2	Q3	Q4
Centre Passes to Goal	24/53=45%	7/14=50%	5/13=36%	7/14=50%	5/12=42%
Restart T/Overs to Goal	12/16=75%	3/3=100%	5/6=83%	1/2=50%	3/5=60%
Live T/Overs to Goal	11/19=58%	2/6=33%	2/3=67%	4/6=67%	3/4=75%
All T/Overs to Goal	23/35=66%	5/9=56%	7/9=78%	5/8=63%	6/9=67%

Figure 6.1 Summary analysis from the netball system.

is that the team only had three live turnovers in each of these two quarters and the coach may have been hoping for a higher number. Similarly, when the team's defence is considered, the coach has not marked opposition restart turnovers in the second quarter even though the opponents scored for all of these. This is because the team only conceded three such turnovers which the coach may feel is acceptable.

Statistics on individual types of turnover can be provided later and trends for these over a series of matches can be monitored. However, immediately after the match, the statistics in Figure 6.1 are enough to start the process of preparing feedback. The combination of two teams' possessions, three possession types (excluding all turnover rows) and four quarters gives 24 fractions and associated percentages to deal with. The selected video sequences are organised into four highlights videos:

- Examples of good attacking play,
- Examples of attacking play where there are areas to improve,
- Examples of good defensive play,
- Examples of defensive play where there are areas to improve.

These highlights videos can be saved as standalone videos to be shared with the squad or individual clips can be saved as separate videos. The two videos on areas for improvement would typically include six clips each. Butterworth (2023a) describes a range of hosting platforms that can be used to share video clips with the squad. These internet-based systems can be accessed by players using their personal devices, allowing engagement with the feedback at times and locations that suit the players' routines. This also allows a greater amount of training time when the squad is together to be devoted to on-court training drills.

The competition schedules in international and domestic netball are different. Some teams had to play seven matches in nine days at the 2023 Netball World Cup. There is typically a week between matches in British National Superleague netball. The match schedules have an impact on the analysis and feedback work done with the squads (Horne, 2013). When matches are played on consecutive days, the squad has limited time for debriefings and briefings. Players may need to take ice baths, eat and sleep. They also do surface practice on match days before the game. Therefore, squad management need to set timetables for each day and ensure squad members have the next day's schedule before the end of the current day.

There is a manual version of the system where possessions played and possessions leading to goals can be tallied. Once the match is over, the totals from the data collection form can be entered into a summary sheet as shown in Figure 6.2. The manual system can be used where an analyst is attending a match not involving their own team, and where it is not possible to access the video recording of the match.

Team		Match:	Opponents	
Goals / Possession	Percentage Conversion	Date:	Goals / Possession	Percentage Conversion
26/51	51%	Centre Passes	26/52	50%
		Turnovers		
12/16	75% great	Interceptions	7/14	50%
7/9	78% great	Sideline balls	1/2	50%
1/7	14% bad	Backline balls	2/9	33% good
3/6	50%	Defensive rebounds	0/2	0%
5/10	50%	Frees / penalties / toss ups	9/16	56% <par
28/48	58% >par	All Turnovers	20/43	46%
15/22	68% great	Turnovers from open play	7/16	44% bad
13/26	50%	Restart turnovers	13/27	46%
55/67	82%	Shooting	46/56	82%
		Rebounds		
2/4		Attacking rebounds taken	3/9	
6/9		Defensive rebounds taken	2/4	

Figure 6.2 Summary sheet for the manual version of the system.

Example 2. UEFA Euro 2022 research

Background and system development

This second example comes from research into women's international soccer (O'Donoghue and Beckley, 2023). The primary purpose of the study was to compare the effectiveness of different types of possession in the UEFA EURO 2022 tournament. There was a secondary purpose to compare the eight quarter-finalists with the eight teams who were eliminated at the end of the group stage. The 31 matches were analysed using a simple code template that was developed in Nacsport Pro (Nacsport, Las Palmas de Gran Canarias, Spain). The code template had six buttons for each team in a match; restart possession start, live possession start, pass, goal, shot on target and shot off target. The full definitions of these events can be found in O'Donoghue and Beckley's (2023) paper. The difference between restart and live possessions is that restart possessions are immediately preceded by a stoppage. Restart possessions include kickoffs, free kicks, throw-ins and corners. Live possessions, on the other hand, commence with one team taking the ball from the other team without any stoppage time between the previous possession and the live possession. These possessions could commence with the ball being intercepted, a successful tackle or a goalkeeper collecting the ball.

This chapter is concerned with the operation of systems once they have already been developed. However, both data collection, data analysis and how results will be presented should all be considered when developing systems. The research had been inspired by Hughes and Frank's (2005) study of possessions in men's World Cup soccer. This compared possessions of different numbers of passes, finding that possessions of five or more passes had a greater chance of leading to shots and goals than possessions of four passes or fewer. Essentially, Hughes and Franks (2005) compared these two types of possession using goals and shots per 1,000 possessions. This avoided presenting misleading findings due to shorter possessions being more common in soccer than longer possessions. To replicate the study of Hughes and Franks (2005) for women's international soccer, O'Donoghue and Beckley (2023) needed to consider whether to code instantaneous events or possessions. Ultimately, the research was comparing possessions of different numbers of passes, so entering possessions during data collection would create data that were in a form ready for statistical analysis. Another advantage of tagging possessions is that whole possessions can be viewed interactively using the system. This would be important if using the system in practical coaching but is not so important in academic research. The disadvantage of tagging possessions is that the number of passes in a possession is not known at the start of the possession. Therefore, separate code buttons for short and long possessions could not be used. It would be possible to use descriptors to add information to coded possessions distinguishing short and long possessions. However, this would require system users to mentally count passes within possessions and add the descriptor after the possession had been completed. An alternative to doing this is to allow individual pass descriptors to be recorded within possessions. Nacsport records the times at which descriptors occur within coded events. This also allows more detailed classification of possessions than a binary choice of long or short. The main reason for not tagging possessions, with passes as descriptors within the possessions, was that it would be easier to tag just passes during data collection if a way could be found to construct possessions from the pass data. This was accomplished by also tagging the start of possessions as instantaneous events. This was to distinguish where two consecutive possessions are performed by the same team. An example of where this can happen is where a team in possession are fouled and, therefore, commence the next possession with a free kick.

Operating environment

The same system was used for all 31 matches and, therefore, no buttons were associated with specific teams. The system had two sets of code buttons; one set was for the "red" team (Team 1) and the other set was for the "blue" team (Team 2). This meant that system operators had to consider one team to be the red team and the other team to be the blue team, even in matches where neither team were wearing red or blue. This was not ideal in a match like the final, where England wore white and Germany wore dark green. However, it did prevent the system having to be altered before each match.

Table 6.1 Replays shown during live ball-in-play time during BBC television coverage of the UEFA Euro 2022 tournament

Match	*Subject of Replay*				
	Attempt on Goal	*Bench or Crowd*	*Live Off the Ball*	*Foul or Alleged Foul*	*Total per 90 mins*
England v Germany*	5	1	0	1	7
France v Holland*	11	2	3	0	16
Sweden v Belgium	2	8	0	0	10
Spain v Denmark	3	0	0	1	4
Austria v Norway	6	1	1	10	18
Portugal v Switzerland	4	3	3	4	14
Iceland v Italy	5	2	1	3	11
N. Ireland v England	4	4	0	0	8
Germany v Finland	3	2	3	0	8
France v Iceland	4	0	4	3	11
Sweden v Holland	5	2	1	1	9
Sweden v Portugal	1	1	2	3	7
Sweden v Switzerland	2	2	0	1	5
England v Sweden	5	0	0	2	7
France v Germany	3	2	0	2	7
France v Italy	6	1	2	0	9
France v Belgium	4	0	0	0	4
Germany v Denmark	4	3	2	1	10
Germany v Spain	4	3	0	0	7
England v Norway	8	1	0	0	9
England v Austria	3	2	0	2	7
Iceland v Belgium	2	2	0	0	4
England v Spain*	6	4	1	2	13
Germany v Austria	7	0	0	3	10
N. Ireland v Austria	4	1	1	4	10
N. Ireland v Norway	7	1	1	0	9
Spain v Finland	4	1	1	1	7
Denmark v Finland	8	2	2	0	12
Holland v Portugal	6	1	0	1	8
Holland v Switzerland	5	2	1	1	9
Belgium v Italy	3	2	0	0	5
Total	144	56	29	46	275

*Match contained extra time.

Data collection was done using match videos allowing videos to be paused when events were being entered. The match videos were from broadcast coverage which contained replays that were occasionally displayed after the match had restarted. There were 275 such replays shown during the coverage of the 31 matches that each prevented at least one possession from being observed. This was equivalent to 8.6 such replays per 90 minute match when one considers that 3 matches included extra time). Therefore, some possessions and passes could not be recorded. Table 6.1 summarises the replays that were shown during live ball-in-play time.

Reliability

The reliability of the process was analysed using an inter-operator agreement study of a full match, once the definitions of events had been agreed by the researchers. This was preceded by a pilot inter-operator agreement study of a 15 minute match section and a discussion of the definitions being used. O'Donoghue and Beckley (2023) describe the reliability study in their paper. This included a cross-tabulation of possessions of different numbers of passes from which a weighted kappa value (Cohen, 1968) was calculated (weighted $\kappa = 0.684$). However, due to restrictions on the length of the paper, the full cross-tabulations of events leading to the kappa values for possession start type and event type could not be included. These two cross-tabulations are shown here in Tables 6.2 and 6.3. There were occasions where a pass was recorded by one of the two researchers but not the other. Indeed, there were occasions where a possession was recorded by one of the observers and not the other. This typically happened where a player contacted the ball and a subjective judgement needed to be made about the level of control the player had over the ball before possession was lost again. The two resulting event lists were exported from Nacsport and needed to be time matched using the process described by O'Donoghue and Holmes (2015: 125–128). This involved entering blank events where one observer did not record anything but the other did (no possession recorded or no event recorded). The time-matched event lists were cross-tabulated using a pivot table in Microsoft Excel. This allowed the kappa values of 0.838 and 0.785 to be determined for possession type and event type respectively (Cohen, 1960).

Table 6.2 Inter-operator agreement for possession type

Observer 1	*Observer 2*					
	Team 1 Live Possession	*Team 1 Restart Possession*	*Team 2 Live Possession*	*Team 2 Restart Possession*	*No Possession Recorded*	*Total*
Team 1 Live Possession	144	1			18	163
Team 1 Restart Possession		57			2	59
Team 2 Live Possession			148	1	19	168
Team 2 Restart Possession			1	59	5	65
No Possession Recorded	3		4	1		8
Total	147	58	153	61	44	463

Table 6.3 Inter-operator agreement for event type within possessions

Observer 1	*Observer 2*					
	Team 1 Pass	*Team 1 Shot*	*Team 2 Pass*	*Team 2 Shot*	*No Event Recorded*	*Total*
Team 1 Pass	674	1			33	708
Team 1 Shot	1	15			1	17
Team 2 Pass			509		48	557
Team 2 Shot				6		6
No Event Recorded	39		39	4		82
Total	714	16	548	10	82	1370

Data processing

The published paper by O'Donoghue and Beckley (2023) lists eight classes of possession based on number of passes and the rate of passes played per second. The definition of high and slow pass rates together with the definitions of live and restart possessions are sufficient to make the methods replicable without going into user manual level detail of the data processing steps used to create the variables. This chapter does describe these steps. In so doing, it is important to discuss the review process of the paper and how this led to the final published version. The paper was initially submitted without analysing the passing rate. The reason for this was to adopt use similar variables to the study of Hughes and Franks (2005) so that differences between women's and men's international soccer could be discussed. This meant that for each team performance in each match, the researchers determined the number of live and restart turnovers of different numbers of passes and the percentage of these that resulted in an attempt on goal. We have already discussed the decision to gather instantaneous events rather than possessions of non-zero duration. The thinking behind this was that if a spreadsheet could be programmed to string passes into possession records, then the functions achieving this could be copied and pasted to apply them to all events gathered from all 31 matches.

Figure 6.3 shows a spreadsheet to determine the number of passes per possession. Columns A to C were taken directly from the event list exported from Nacsport. Events performed by Team 1 and Team 2 had been tagged using red and blue buttons in the code template, respectively. The first thing the researchers needed to do was transform the event into separate columns for the team performing the event and the event type. This was essential to eventually use pivot tables to produce summary records for the two teams within the match. This was done in columns D and E. The cells D2 and E2 contain the Excel expressions shown in Equations 6.1 and 6.2, respectively. Cell D2 was relatively easy to program. The researchers knew the team was either "Team 1" or "Team 2" and so this could be determined from the coded event in cell B2 using a simple text processing function (LEFT). Determining the event type was a little harder because the event types have differing numbers of characters. These characters were to the RIGHT of cell B2 and the number of characters was the LENgth of the string minus seven to remove the team name and the space that separated the team and the event type.

$$=\text{LEFT}(\text{B2,6}) \tag{6.1}$$

$$=\text{RIGHT}(\text{B2,LEN}(\text{B2})-7) \tag{6.2}$$

The "Pass Error" column was used during data cleaning to identify potentially incorrect data, for example, a live turnover where the team was the same as the team performing the previous event. The length of possessions in column I is the number of passes within the possession. The number of passes is only included in this column once a possession ends. In this way, the spreadsheet contains a row for each instantaneous event (start of a possession, pass, shot or goal), but column I reduces this to possession level data by leaving cells blank where possessions have not been completed. The process of producing the number of passes per possession (column I) requires us to accumulate passes made within possessions; this is done in column G. The cell G5 contains the Excel expression shown in Equation 6.3. This uses nested IF functions because there are three things that can happen in column G. Firstly, this may be the start of a new possession with the first pass still having to be played. This situation is recognised if the left most characters of event type (column E) spell "Possession". In this situation, we have 0 passes so far within the possession. The second thing that could happen is that the row contains data for a pass. If this is the case, then the event type (column E) will be "Pass" and the number of passes so far will simply be one more than it was in the previous row. The third thing that can happen is that something other than a pass occurs within a possession. This could be a shot or a goal. Hence, the else part of the inner IF statement simply copies the number of passes played so far from the previous row. Having determined the number of passes played within possessions and setting this back to zero when a new possession commences (column G), it is relatively simple to produce column I. This is done using the Excel expression shown in Equation 6.4 which is for the cell I5. This basically looks at the next row to see if it is starting a new possession, and if it is, then the current row must be ending the possession. Hence, the number of passes played so far in the possession is simply copied from column G to column I. Where the next row is not starting a new possession, column I simply contains an empty character string.

$$=\text{IF}(\text{RIGHT}(\text{E5,10})=\text{"Possession",0,IF}(\text{E5="Pass",G4+1,G4}))) \tag{6.3}$$

$$=\text{IF}(\text{RIGHT}(\text{E6,10})=\text{"Possession",G5,""}) \tag{6.4}$$

The final thing to do is determine the type of possession and ensure this is stored in the same row as the number of passes in the possession. As you can see

	A	B	C	D	E	F	G	H	I
1	N#	Category	Click	Team	Event	Pass Error	Possession length so far	Possession type	Length
2	1	Team 2 Restart Possession	03:09	Team 2	Restart Possession		0	Restart Possession	
3	1	Team 2 Pass	03:21	Team 2	Pass		1	Restart Possession	
4	2	Team 2 Pass	03:22	Team 2	Pass		2	Restart Possession	2
5	1	Team 1 Restart Possession	03:30	Team 1	Restart Possession		0	Restart Possession	
6	1	Team 1 Pass	03:44	Team 1	Pass		1	Restart Possession	
7	2	Team 1 Pass	03:49	Team 1	Pass		2	Restart Possession	
8	3	Team 1 Pass	03:50	Team 1	Pass		3	Restart Possession	
9	4	Team 1 Pass	03:52	Team 1	Pass		4	Restart Possession	
10	5	Team 1 Pass	03:53	Team 1	Pass		5	Restart Possession	5
11	1	Team 2 Live Possession	03:57	Team 2	Live Possession		0	Live Possession	
12	3	Team 2 Pass	03:59	Team 2	Pass		1	Live Possession	1
13	1	Team 1 Live Possession	04:00	Team 1	Live Possession		0	Live Possession	
14	6	Team 1 Pass	04:02	Team 1	Pass		1	Live Possession	
15	7	Team 1 Pass	04:07	Team 1	Pass		2	Live Possession	
16	8	Team 1 Pass	04:12	Team 1	Pass		3	Live Possession	3
17	2	Team 2 Live Possession	04:15	Team 2	Live Possession		0	Live Possession	
18	4	Team 2 Pass	04:15	Team 2	Pass		1	Live Possession	1
19	2	Team 1 Live Possession	04:18	Team 1	Live Possession		0	Live Possession	

Figure 6.3 Spreadsheet to determine number of passes per possession.

in column H, blanks are not used in the cells prior to the possession completing. This is because when column I is eventually used with columns D and H, we can ignore any values from columns D and H that are associated with blank cells from column H. Column H determines the possession type at the start of a possession and copies this into each row until the possession ends. This is done using the Excel expression in Equation 6.5 which is for the cell H5.

$$=\text{IF}\left(\text{RIGHT}\left(\text{E5,10}\right)=\text{"Possession",E5,H4}\right) \tag{6.5}$$

It is also necessary to include additional columns to determine whether possessions led to shots or not. This is done using a similar approach of checking if there was a shot so far within a possession and then using this at the end of the possession. If this were to be added in column J, then we would have the Excel expression shown in Equation 6.6 in cell J5. This is another example of where one of three things could happen. First, the row could represent the start of a new possession where a shot has not been observed yet and so we simply set the cell to "No" meaning no shot so far. Second, if the event (column E) is a "Shot on target", "Shot off target" or a "Goal", then we want to set the cell to "Yes" meaning that a shot has been recorded within the possession. Note the use of the LEFT function so we can simply ask about shot rather than distinguishing shots on target from shots off target. The third thing that can happen is that the current row is within a possession but a shot is not taking place; the row could simply be a pass within the possession. In this situation, whether a shot has occurred within the possession or not does not change from the previous row. Hence, the contents of the cell J4 are simply copied into J5.

$$\begin{aligned}&=\text{IF}\left(\text{RIGHT}\left(\text{E5,10}\right)=\text{"Possession","No",IF}\left(\text{OR}\left(\text{E5}\right.\right.\right.\\&\quad\left.\left.\left.=\text{"Goal",LEFT}\left(\text{E5,4}\right)=\text{"Shot"}\right),\text{"Yes", J4}\right)\right)\end{aligned} \tag{6.6}$$

Exercise: As an exercise, how would you change Equation 6.6 if you wanted to classify possessions as leading to "Goal", "Shot on target", "Shot off target" or "No shot"? Try this for the cell J5. You will find the answer at the end of this chapter in Equation 6.12.

As mentioned previously, the concept of passing rate was introduced into the paper at the suggestion of the reviewers. In order to determine the pass rate, it was necessary to determine the duration of the possessions in seconds and then combine with the number of passes. This required the spreadsheet to note the start time of the possession and copy this into the remaining rows for the possession so that it would be available at the end of the possession to be subtracted from the end time for the possession. The time of an event is represented in a Nacsport event list as shown in column C of Figure 6.3 (Click). This is a video time in minutes and seconds; so, 101:20 would represent 101 minutes 20 s into the match video. The total number of seconds into the video is determined to facilitate arithmetic processing of the times. This is done using text processing in Excel. Firstly, we need to determine where the colon is within the character string that represents the video time. If this was done in column K of the spreadsheet, then cell K5 would contain the Excel expression shown in Equation 6.7. Having determined the location of the colon and presented this in cell K5, we can now use this along with Nacsport representation of video time in C5 to produce the total number of seconds as shown in Equation 6.8. This Excel expression is in the cell L5. Note the addition of 0 to the number of minutes and to the number of seconds. This is because the text processing functions LEFT and RIGHT produce text strings such as "101" and "20" which are different to the numeric values 101 and 20. However, by adding zero, a value of a numeric type, Excel evaluates the two sub-expressions into values of numeric types. Thus, we will get an overall value of 6080 as the time in seconds corresponding to the Nacsport representation 101:20.

$$=\text{FIND}(\text{":"},\text{C5}) \tag{6.7}$$

$$=\left(\text{LEFT}(\text{C5},\text{K5-1})+0\right)^{*}60+\text{RIGHT}\left(\text{C5},\text{LEN}(\text{C5})-\text{K5}\right)+0 \tag{6.8}$$

Once this was done, the cells in columns D to L could be pasted down for the remaining rows in a spreadsheet that contained all of the events for all 31 matches. Additional columns were added to represent the actual teams within the matches as three letter codes. For example, "ENG" and "GER" were used for England and Germany. This permitted a series of data reduction steps to be applied to produce a data sheet suitable to be uploaded into a statistics package. These steps are listed below:

- The event level data were transformed into performance data using a pivot table. There were over 40,000 events within the 31 matches. These data were reduced to 62 performances because there were two teams contesting each match. The pivot table had a row for each performance and then clustered columns for possession type (this was a composite variable based on how the possession started, the number of passes and the pass rate) and outcome (shot or no shot).

- Team data were then aggregated. Some teams played three matches because they were eliminated at the end of the group stage while England and Germany played six matches because they reached the final. The aggregated data had a row for each of the 16 teams containing the variables for their average performance (using the mean for each variable from the set of matches they played in). There were three matches, and hence six team performances, where extra time was played. The frequency data from these matches was scaled by a factor of 0.75 before contributing to the aggregated performance for the given team.
- The final step was to include a team type variable to distinguish the eight quarter-finalists from the eight teams eliminated at the end of the group stage.

Statistical analysis

There is not much to add about statistical analysis that has not already been published in the paper (O'Donoghue and Beckley, 2023). Normality was checked using Shapiro Wilk tests rather than Kolmogorov Smirnov tests because there were fewer than 50 values for each variable once the data had been reduced to the aggregated records for each team. Medians, lower and upper quartiles were used as descriptive statistics given that the data were not normally distributed. Nonparametric tests were used to compare the two types of teams (Mann-Whitney U tests), productivity of live and restart possessions (Wilcoxon signed-ranks tests) and the productivity of possessions of different lengths and passing rates (Friedman tests).

The one thing that does require more coverage in this text book is the calculation of Cliff's delta as an effect size. The paper has stated that this was used and what values are interpreted as small (0.11), moderate (0.28) and large effects (0.43). This is sufficient to make the methods replicable in this respect because Cliff's delta, like any other existing statistical procedure, can be looked up from elsewhere without the paper having to "re-invent the wheel". The same might be said of this text book. However, a purpose of text books is to bring together detail of various tasks that students may need to perform.

Cliff's delta is an effect size that can be used with ordinal, interval or ratio scale data, making it suitable for use with nonparametric inferential statistics. We will use the percentage of restart possessions that led to attempts on goal as an example. Table 6.4 shows the values for this variable for the two types of teams. Each value from the first group (quarter-finalists) is compared with each value from the second group (eliminated teams) to determine the direction of the differences in the M × N difference. Here, the two groups are the same size with M and N both being 8, but this is not always the case. The direction of the difference is +1 if the value from the first group is greater than that of the second group, −1 if it is smaller and 0 if the two values are the same. This allows an M × N (8 × 8) grid of direction scores to be determined as shown in Table 6.5. An Excel spreadsheet can be programmed to determine the direction values in a two-dimensional table using nested

Table 6.4 The percentage of restart possessions that led to attempts on goal

Quarter-Finalists	*Teams Eliminated After the Group Stage*
6.38	3.94
2.24	2.02
11.16	3.30
6.24	7.29
2.29	2.44
9.72	4.37
12.37	3.17
4.58	2.51

Table 6.5 Direction scores between each value from the quarter-finalists and each value from the eliminated teams

Quarter-Finalist Values	*Teams Eliminated After the Group Stage*							
	3.94	*2.02*	*3.30*	*7.29*	*2.44*	*4.37*	*3.17*	*2.51*
6.38	+1	+1	+1	−1	+1	+1	+1	+1
2.24	−1	+1	−1	−1	−1	−1	−1	−1
11.16	+1	+1	+1	+1	+1	+1	+1	+1
6.24	+1	+1	+1	−1	+1	+1	+1	+1
2.29	−1	+1	−1	−1	−1	−1	−1	−1
9.72	+1	+1	+1	+1	+1	+1	+1	+1
12.37	+1	+1	+1	+1	+1	+1	+1	+1
4.58	+1	+1	+1	−1	+1	+1	+1	+1

IF functions. If you use absolute addressing ($) correctly within one of these cells, it can be pasted into the remaining cells yielding the correct values. The sum of these values is determined using Equation 6.9, where M is the number of values in the first sample, N is the number of values in the second sample, i represents the ith value in the first sample, and j represents the jth value in the second sample.

$$delta = \frac{1}{MN}\sum_{i=1}^{M}\sum_{j=1}^{N} direction(i, j) \qquad (6.9)$$

In our example, the sum of the direction scores is 30. This is divided by 64 (8×8) to give a Cliff's delta value of 0.47 which is interpreted as a large effect.

Quantitative research

The research used as an example in this section of the paper (O'Donoghue and Beckley, 2023) was a quantitative research study where matches were abstracted to a fingerprint of quantitative variables and then presented for broad groups of teams: the average quarter-finalist, the average team eliminated at the end of the group stage or the average team within the tournament. This subsection of the current chapter discusses some concerns about this traditional reductive way of undertaking quantitative research. The paper concluded that possessions of five or more passes with a slow pass rate were the most productive for generating attempts on goal. However, the paper also acknowledged that this conclusion did not apply to all teams. There were six of the 16 teams for whom possessions of nine or more passes with a slow pass rate were not the most productive for creating scoring opportunities. Restart possessions of one or two passes were the most productive for three of the teams, possessions of five to eight passes with a slow pass rate were the most productive for two others, with one team having their highest percentage of attempts on goal from restart possessions of three or four passes. Figure 6.4 shows the percentage of short and long possessions that led to attempts on goal for each team in the Euro 2022 tournament. This does not distinguish between restart or live possessions, or between possessions with high and low passing rates. The grey band running from bottom left to top right represents teams who generate attempts on goal from a similar percentage of these two broad types of possession. Teams like Denmark and Sweden would be advised

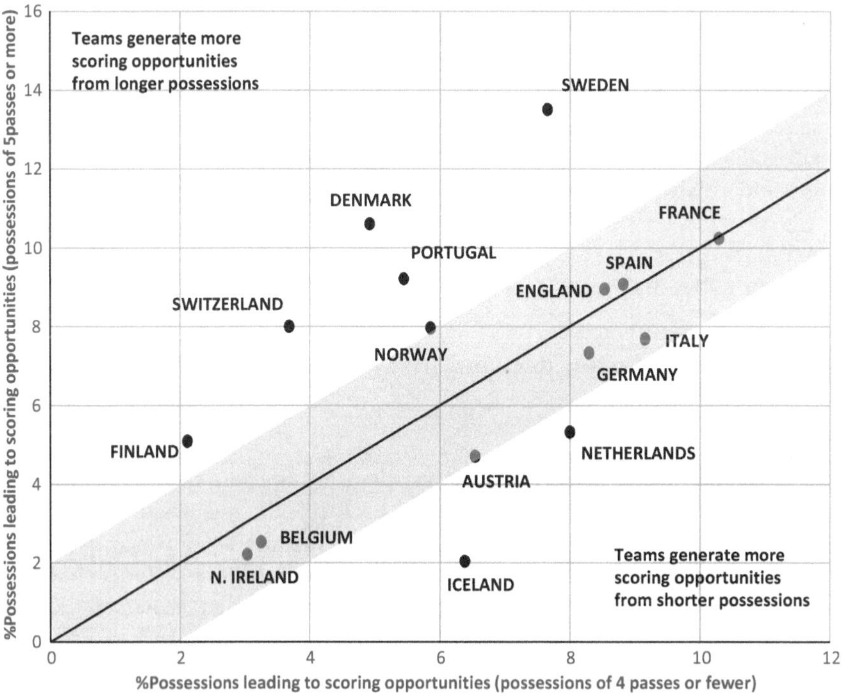

Figure 6.4 The percentage of possessions leading to scoring opportunities for different teams in the Euro 2022 soccer tournament.

to adopt a more elaborate possession style because this appears to be more productive for these teams than using a more direct style of play. Iceland, on the other hand, produce scoring opportunities from a greater percentage of shorter possessions that characterise a more direct style of play.

What may surprise readers about Figure 6.4 is that it suggests Spain are just as productive from shorter possessions as they are from longer possessions. They are considered to be a team that uses a "tiki taka" style of play and Spain's possessions contain more passes than the other teams in the tournament. So why are longer possessions not more productive for Spain? We will consider one of Spain's shots on target from their group match against Finland. The shot was taken around 47:45, that is in the third minute of the second half. Spain had a possession of 14 passes where they moved the ball up the field and played the ball into the penalty area. The ball was headed away by a Finnish defender, with a second Finnish defender also playing the ball in the air. The fact that a header (counted as a headed pass in the research study) went to a teammate, meant that this was counted as a live possession for Finland. However, the second header went to a Spanish player to start a new possession for Spain which consisted of two passes followed by a shot on goal from outside the penalty area. Given the definitions being used in the research study, this shot on target was deemed to have come from a short possession of two passes. However, when viewing the video, there is evidence that the previous possession of 14 passes led to the ball being in the attacking third and making a contribution to the shot on goal, even though Finland had a couple of touches of the ball in between. There are many examples in soccer where an elaborate possession leads to territorial advantage such that even if the defending team temporarily takes possession of the ball, they can lose the ball again under pressure leading to a goal being conceded. This highlights an issue with objectivity, operational definitions and restricting analysts from using experience and expertise when collecting data.

Example 3. Analysing decision making

Background and development

The third example is a system to analyse decision making during Australian Rules football performance (Lorains et al., 2013). This is not a system that the authors have experience of using but is being used as an example here for several reasons. Firstly, the previous two examples are systems that the authors have used which means that there is a possibility that some issues may not have been raised simply because they are things the authors take for granted as experienced users of the systems. Discussing a system developed by others gives greater scope for questioning meanings and processes. The authors of this book do have some experience in analysing decision making because a current PhD researcher at Cardiff Metropolitan University is investigating decision making during fast break situations in women's basketball. The second reason for using this system is to analyse decision making where more variables require analyst expertise and training to record reliably. Thirdly, decision making is an important area; the authors of the paper described decision making as an important but largely ignored area in sports performance analysis. Ten years on from the publication of their paper, there has been further research in the area (Lima e Silva et al., 2020; Machado et al., 2020, 2023; Miarka et al., 2016), but it remains an area requiring much more research. Fourthly, it is fair to say that the variables in the previous two examples are more matter-of-fact than some of the variables in this third example. It is very important that one of the examples used in this chapter contains variables that are less matter-of-fact so that the challenges in analysing these can be discussed. A fifth reason for using this example is that it has been used in both practically in a coaching environment and in research that has led to publication (Lorains et al., 2013).

The system was implemented in Microsoft Excel. Figure 6.5 shows the variables in Lorains et al.'s (2013) system and their possible values. This representation of the system does not include some on-screen areas that show currently selected values and provides a button to confirm and register the current event. The events recorded using the system are occasions where a player receives the ball and needs to "consciously dispose" of the ball. The ball is usually disposed of by a hand pass or kicking the ball into space or to a teammate.

This example, like the previous example, uses broadcast coverage. The footage was provided by the broadcaster and included both side-on and end-on views. It is not clear if this means that the footage as shown to viewers was used (which would include different views at different times) or if the recordings from each angle were provided for the full match duration of each match. If all of the footage from all angles are provided, as recorded, it also avoids the replays being shown. The use of multiple views of the same events can potentially improve accuracy but increases the time required to enter data.

Operating environment

The human operation of the system is part of the system and so the system was developed, operators trained for five weeks to use it, tested for reliability and amended if necessary. We will discuss reliability of the system as we cover the different variables. Figure 6.5 shows that the system is well laid out so that the left to right arrangement of buttons reflects the order with which operators enter data. The use of Microsoft Excel means that the video is not being indexed directly and, hence, the reason why the time of events needs to be entered. The general information about the time and location of the ball reception will be known as soon as the player received the ball. The next set of variables are for decision making and require repeated viewing of events,

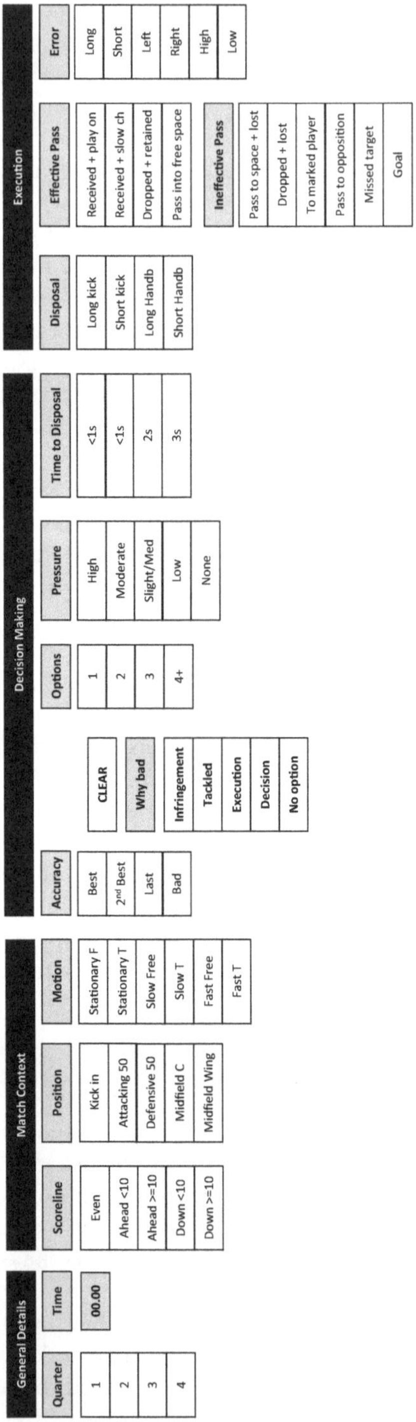

Figure 6.5 A system to analyse decision-making performance in Australian Rules football (adapted from Lorains et al., 2013).

possibly pausing and playing at half speed. The time to disposal is straightforward and can be derived from the video clock. The pressure the player was under and the number of options that were realistically available are ordinal variables that require expert knowledge of the sport. The easiest situation is if there are four or more options because the operator does not distinguish these situations. Greater thought is needed if there are one or two options or two or three options.

There is an interesting point about judging the number of options available to players. A system like this could be used differently by different analysts for quite legitimate reasons. A squad may have a particular philosophy or a particular way of playing which dictates, to a certain extent, what players should do in different situations. For example, high performance squads may have shared mental models that enhance co-ordination (Ashford et al., 2023). Others may use the system, considering all available options rather than those dictated by a particular style of play. The research being done in basketball by one of the authors of this book analyses pressure differently from how Lorains et al. (2013) have done for Australian Rules football. Lorains et al.'s (2013) system uses five alternative values for pressure which means there is more scope for disagreement between operators than if pressure was high, moderate and low with low including situations where the observers perceive there to be no pressure on the player.

The use of a shared mental model by the squad may also help the analysts in classifying the accuracy of the system. There may be occasions where there is a particular option that should be chosen that would be considered the best option. Where there is no shared mental model or where the analysts are not aware of a shared mental model being applied, the classification of decision accuracy is more difficult. Some research has used the outcome of the event as an indication of decision accuracy (Bruce et al., 2009). If this were being done, then there actually would not be any need for a separate variable for decision accuracy. Lorains et al. (2013) make an excellent justification for separating the accuracy of the decision from the outcome of the event. There are occasions in sport where a player makes a good decision but the execution of the chosen option results in an unsuccessful outcome. For example, a soccer player may attempt a penetrative pass that has a chance of being intercepted but which may lead to a scoring opportunity for a teammate if the ball reaches the teammate. Whether or not the decision to attempt the penetrative pass was an accurate decision depends on a number of factors. Firstly, there is the perceived probability of the pass being successful. This should not only be considered for the specific event being observed but also needs to consider the overall choice to use such an option in similar situations within the match. It could be that the penetrative pass has a probability of success that is less than 0.25. However, if this type of pass is attempted enough times, it will lead to scoring opportunities being created. Secondly, the consequences of the penetrative pass being unsuccessful in the specific situation need to be considered. Such passes may be attempted in order to generate some scoring opportunities during the match. However is a particular situation, attempting such a pass may be considered to be a poor option as teammates may be poorly positioned to deal with an opposition counterattack. Indeed, if such a penetrative pass actually does lead to a scoring opportunity, it might be considered a poor decision even though there was a successful outcome. Thirdly, it may be necessary to consider the player's awareness of the available options. The analyst might see four options but might rule two of these out if they believe the player could not have been aware of them from where the player was situated or the pressure the player was under. Thus, the best decision of those the players was aware of might be different to the best decision of all of the options the analyst can see. On the other hand, the analyst may feel that the player should have been aware of all available options. For example, visual scanning can be used by players throughout the match so that they are better prepared to receive the ball and successfully dispose of it (Aksum et al., 2021).

The final set of variables are concerned with execution once the player has chosen an option. Lorains et al. (2013) describe this as the execution of the disposal of the ball. However, in some sports, players may have choices about how they receive the ball and some of these options may be better than others. A player may decide to take a ball in the air or allow the ball to bounce before collecting it. They may decide to hold position, shielding the area where they will collect the ball, rather than moving towards the ball. They may have the option to catch the ball or play the ball with a single touch with hand(s) or feet. This can potentially make the assessment of execution quite complicated if an event can be broken down into different parts such as collecting the ball, movement and disposing of the ball. Using separate variables for the execution of these different elements of the event could over-complicate the information being provided in feedback to players. Similarly, if the system were being used in a descriptive research study, the results may become over-complex if execution is decomposed in this way. Thus, using and applying the execution variables to the overall event or to a particular part of the event may lead to a more concise and manageable presentation of results. The guidance given by Lorains et al. (2013) to analyse the execution of the disposal enhances the clarity of the system and the information it produces. The way in which the ball is disposed of and the effectiveness of this are reasonably straightforward. This is because the analyst is not required to make judgements about the relative opportunities and risks of different options at this point. They are simply recording what the player did and what happened next. For each event, they will select one of the values for an effective pass or one of the values for an ineffective disposal. The final variable to be entered is the nature of any error made during the execution of the disposal. There is a possibility that an ineffective disposal may be played too high and too short. The system could be implemented in a way that allows any errors that apply in a situation to be recorded. However, if this system is implemented in Microsoft Excel using a single column to record the effectiveness of execution, then the operator will need to select the primary error class that applies.

Calculating reliability statistics

The previous subsection discussed the challenges in recording the very important variables that are included in the system. In so doing, the previous subsection also discussed the potentially limited reliability of the system. Lorains et al. (2013) have reported the reliability levels of the different variables in their system. The kappa values range from 0.79 for the number of options to 0.98 for time in the match which may be more matter of fact. This subsection will use number of options and disposal as example variables to show how reliability statistics can be calculated. We do not have access to the data of Lorains et al. (2013) but use fictitious frequencies of values to illustrate how to calculate reliability.

Disposal is a nominal variable because we have no reason for saying hand passes are better or worse than kicking the ball, and no reason for considering long or short passes to be superior. Inter-operator agreement for such a nominal variable can be calculated using the kappa statistic (Cohen, 1960). Table 6.6 shows the agreements and disagreements between two fictitious trained operators. Here, we assume that the operators agree that there are 294 events where a player receives the ball and consciously attempts to dispose of it. We are also assuming that the same 294 events are recorded by each operator. This makes the evaluation of reliability simpler than the Euro 2022 passing example. The cells on the top left to bottom right diagonal contain the 271 events where the two operators agree on the disposal. There are some understandable disagreements where the length of a kick (or hand pass) may be on the threshold between what would be considered short and long. It would actually be surprising if such disagreements did not exist. What is of greater concern is the five events where the operators disagree about whether a disposal was a kick or a hand pass. There is one of these where they disagree on the length of the disposal as well.

The kappa statistic calculates the proportion of agreements excluding any agreements that the operators could have achieved by chance. The raw proportion of agreements, P_0, is 0.9218 (= 271/294). Some agreements could have been achieved by one or both of the operators guessing the disposal type. Operator 1 recorded 55 long kicks. Knowing that Operator 2 has recorded 49 long kicks out of 294 events tells us that there is a 49/294 probability

Table 6.6 Agreements and disagreements between two independent operators for the disposal variable

Operator 1	*Operator 2*				
	Long Kick	*Short Kick*	*Long Hand Pass*	*Short Hand Pass*	*Total*
Long kick	46	8	1	0	55
Short kick	3	87	0	2	92
Long hand pass	0	1	12	5	18
Short hand pass	0	1	2	126	129
Total	49	97	15	133	294

of agreeing with Operator 2 that the event is a long kick when Operator 1 guesses that it is long kick. Multiplying this fraction by the 55 occasions where Operator 1 has recorded a long kick gives an expected number of agreements by guessing of 9.1667 (= 55 × 49/294) for long kick. Applying this to the remaining values gives expected numbers of agreements of 30.3537, 0.9184, and 58.3571 for short kick, long hand pass and short hand pass, respectively. Summing these gives a total expected number of agreements by chance of 98.7959. Thus, the probability of agreeing by chance, P_C, is 0.3360 (= 98.7959/294). To exclude the probability of agreeing by chance, we consider P_0 to be itself divided by 1. Kappa, κ, is calculated by subtracting P_C from the dividend and divisor of this division as shown in Equation 6.10. This gives a kappa value of 0.8822.

$$\kappa = \left(P_0 - P_C\right) / \left(1 - P_C\right) \tag{6.10}$$

Altman (1991: 404) interprets kappa values of 0.8 and over as representing a very good strength of agreement. The strength of agreement is considered good if kappa is at least 0.6 but less than 0.8, moderate if at least 0.4 but less than 0.6, fair if at least 0.2 but less than 0.4, otherwise poor if less than 0.2. These threshold values come from applied medical research and so the threshold values used in sports performance analysis may need to differ. For example, in work-rate analysis, a kappa value of 0.8 or above could be considered good, a value of at least 0.5 but less than 0.8 is acceptable, but values of less than 0.5 would be considered poor (O'Donoghue, 2015: 200–206).

Number of options is an ordinal variable where we could use the weighted version of kappa (Cohen, 1968). The advantage of weighted kappa is that slight disagreements, for example, between 1 and 2 options, are considered differently to serious disagreements, for example, between 1 and 4+ options. Table 6.7 shows the agreements and disagreements for two fictitious operators for the number of options. The unweighted kappa statistic that was used for disposal would be 0.7168 if applied to the number of options. If checking this as an exercise, you should get 0.8367 and 0.4235 for P_0 and P_C, respectively.

When we calculate weighted kappa, the agreements as well as the agreements expected by chance include where credit is given for minor disagreements. In

Table 6.7 Agreements and disagreements between two independent operators for the number of options

Operator 1	*Operator 2*				
	1	*2*	*3*	*4+*	*Total*
1	17	2	0	0	19
2	4	51	17	1	73
3	0	14	154	7	175
4+	0	0	3	24	27
Total	21	67	174	32	294

Table 6.8 Weights used in the calculation of weighted kappa for the number of options

Operator 1	*Operator 2*			
	1	*2*	*3*	*4+*
1	1	0.5	0	0
2	0.5	1	0.5	0
3	0	0.5	1	0.5
4+	0	0	0.5	1

this example, we count disagreements between 1 and 2, 2 and 3, 3 and 4+ as 0.5 of an agreement. The use of 0.5 is an arbitrary weight and we could have used 0.25 or some other number between 0 and 1. The weight depends on how serious we consider the disagreement to be; 0.25 would be used where disagreements are more serious and 0.5 where disagreements are less serious. Table 6.8 shows the weights being used in this example.

The calculation of P_0 for weighted kappa uses all 16 cells of the cross-tabulation of frequencies and not just the cells on the top left to bottom right diagonal. Let N be our total of 294 events. Our variable, number of options, has 4 values. We will use V to represent the number of values. Equation 6.11 is used to calculate the weighted number of agreements, where $f_{i,j}$ is the frequency of events where Operator 1 records the ith value for the variable and Operator 2 records the jth value (i and j can take the values 1, 2, 3 or 4). Also, $w_{i,j}$ represents the weight given where Operator 1 records the ith value for the variable and Operator 2 records the jth value (these weights are seen in Table 6.8). Where the weight is 1 for a complete agreement about the number of options, the actual frequency is used. For example, the 51 occasions where the two operators agreed that there were 2 options. Where there is a weight of 0.5, the frequency is multiplied by this weight. For example, 8.5 is used for the 17 occasions where Operator 1 recorded 2 options but Operator 2 recorded 3. Consider the one occasion where Operator 1 recorded 2 options but Operator 2 recorded 4+. A weight of 0 here means that this will not contribute to the weighted agreements. Applying Equation 6.11 to the frequencies in Table 6.7 and the weights in Table 6.8 gives us a total of 269.5. Hence, weighted P_0 is 0.9167 when we divide by 294 (N).

$$Weighted\ \ agreements = \sum_{i=1}^{V} \sum_{j=1}^{V} w_{i,j} f_{i,j} \tag{6.11}$$

When we calculated the number of agreements we could expect by chance, we summed the expected number of agreements by chance for each of the 4 values of the variable. When using the weighted version of kappa, the expected number of agreements by chance needs to be calculated for partial agreements as well as complete agreements. The 73 occasions where Operator 1 recorded that there were two options. Knowing that Operator 2 recorded 3 options on

174 occasions tells us there is a probability of 174/294 that there will be a partial agreement between 2 and 3 options when Operator 1 guesses there are 2 options. Multiplying this by the number of occasions where Operator 1 recorded 2 options gives an expected number of partial agreements between 2 options for Operator 1 and 3 options for Operator 2 of 43.2041 (= 73 × 174/294). Basically, to work out the number of partial agreements between any pair of values for the number of options, we simply consider the cell, multiply the row total from Table 6.7 by the column total from Table 6.7 and divide this by N (the grand total of 294). Now, because this is a partial agreement, we need to multiply this expected frequency by the weight of 0.5 to get 21.6020 contributing to the weighted agreements by chance. Doing this for all 16 cells of the cross-tabulated frequencies with corresponding weights gives a total of 188.3316 agreements by guessing including partial agreements. This is divided by N (294) to give a probability of 0.6406 of an agreement or partial agreement by guessing. We can now apply Equation 6.10 to our proportion of agreements and partial agreements ($P_0 = 0.9167$) and our proportion of agreements and partial agreements, we would expect by chance ($P_C = 0.6406$) to achieve a weighted kappa value of 0.7681. So in this example, using the weighted version of kappa has given a higher value than the unweighted version by giving credit for partial agreements. Sometimes, weighted kappa can give a lower value than the unweighted kappa statistic because it adds to the P_C term as well as the P_0 term of kappa.

Use in research

The main purpose of the research study done by Lorains et al. (2013) was to compare decision accuracy of a set of 13 players between early and late season games and thus evaluate the effectiveness of a five-week video-based decision-making training intervention that the players engaged with. The players were awarded points between 0 and 3 for the quality of the decisions made during ball reception and disposal events. The pooled frequencies of decision scores for the 13 players were compared between the two early season matches and the two late season matches. This revealed that the percentage of events where decision quality achieved the top mark of 3 points increased from 39% in the early season matches to 64% in the late season matches. They also reported that this improvement in decision making was achieved despite the pressure players were under and the number of options they had available being similar between the early and late season matches.

This subsection considers additional analyses that could be conducted with the data gathered using this system. Any analysis should be dictated by the purpose of the study and researchers should avoid a multivariate data grubbing approach of analysing every pair of variables within this set of variables. Potential research questions include:

- Does the level a player plays at influence decision-making performance in the given sport,
- Does scoreline influence decision-making performance,

- Does match period (quarter or half) influence decision-making performance,
- Do winning teams within matches have different decision-making performance to losing teams.

When investigating these questions, decision-making performance is a set of dependent variables including the number of options available to players, the percentage of time they find themselves under different levels of pressure, time to disposal, the accuracy of their decisions and the percentage of time where there was an effective execution of the chosen option rather than an ineffective execution. The number of options is not strictly a numerical variable due to the 4+ category. Therefore, it may need to be transformed into a score or divided into four separate variables for the percentage of times players have 1, 2, 3 or 4+ options. Pressure could also be converted into a score. Time to disposal is based on the terminology used in Lorains et al.'s (2013) study of Australian Rules football. More generally, this would be the time to take a decision. This may be important if the accuracy of decisions is not significantly influenced by any independent variable, but decisions are made quicker in some situations than in others. The match context variables may need to be controlled for if some players perform in different areas of the pitch or if they start with different motions to other players. This would be especially needed if decision-making dependent variables differed between these different contexts for events.

Associations between the decision-making variables is also an important area of research. If we are looking at relationships between number of options and decision accuracy, it may be necessary to exclude any events where there is only one option if we assume the player will choose the only option available to them and this is considered the best option. The accuracy of decision and the technical execution of the chosen option may be considered to be independent elements of performance. Nonetheless, it is an interesting research question to compare technical execution between situations where the best, second best, last and bad options are chosen.

You may have noticed that the research questions we have discussed do not go into different types of disposal or different types of effective and ineffective disposal. There may be valid and important research questions you can think of that include these variables. There is a point about research design that we wish to make here. If a system is being developed for a research study, it should not include variables that are not going to be used. Entering additional variables takes time, causes operator fatigue and may lower the level of reliability for the important variables that are actually going to be analysed.

Use in practice

Lorains et al. (2013) implemented the system in Microsoft Excel. However, the system could also be implemented using a commercial video analysis package. This could include an additional variable for player performing the event allowing any players who need to improve their decision making to be identified. The data for these players could then be explored to determine if there are any types of situation, periods of matches or contextual factors associated with less accurate decisions being made. Combinations of these can then be used when interacting with matrices of situations and decision-making parameters to view related video sequences. This allows coaches and players to look in greater depth at potential causes of inaccurate decisions being made. Such information and discussions about these findings can help tailor coaching advice and training activities to improve decision-making performance.

Answer to exercise

Earlier in this chapter, we gave you an exercise to change Equation 6.6 so that it would determine the outcomes of possessions using more than two values. Equation 6.12 shows an answer but there are other ways of doing this. By changing the inner IF to deal with passes in the then part rather than the else part, we can simply use the contents of column E in Figure 6.3 to set the value for any row that is not the start of a possession or a pass. This will either be a goal, shot on target or shot off target.

$$= \text{IF}\left(\text{RIGHT}\left(\text{E5,10}\right)=\text{"Possession","No shot",IF}\left(\text{LEFT}\left(\text{E5,4}\right)\right.\right.$$
$$\left.\left.=\text{"Pass"},\text{J4},\text{E5}\right)\right) \tag{6.12}$$

Conclusion

This chapter has discussed the analysis of coded match data using examples from three different scenarios; one from coaching, one from academic research and the third which combines research and practice. The purpose of the analysis coaching and research scenarios is different. In coaching, data are analysed to produce statistical and video feedback to help players improve. The time scale for this type of analysis is dictated by match schedules and when information is needed to inform training. The timescale for analysing data for academic research is longer because the research paper can be submitted at any time to a scientific journal as long as the research is still current. There are similarities in the analysis work that is done in coaching and research contexts. Firstly, reliability of data is important in both contexts and steps are taken to detect and correct errors as far as possible as well as acknowledge any remaining limits of reliability. Secondly, data from video analysis packages are exported to other packages for processing in order to produce higher order summary statistics.

7 Sports video telestration

Introduction

Video telestration is a technique that is commonly used in television broadcasting and has revolutionised the way sports broadcasters analyse and visualise key moments of a match. The technique involves the use of computer vision technology to superimpose freehand annotations or graphics over video footage, providing in-depth insight into sports events and a more engaging viewing experience (Thomas et al., 2017). The 'telestrator', or the magic crayon, as it was dubbed, was reportedly first used on 3 January 1982 by legendary American football coach and commentator John Madden during the National Football League (NFL) play-off game between New York Giants and San Francisco 49ers live on CBS (Slate, 2018). Using visual annotations and expert commentary, Madden used the 'telestrator' to breakdown the 49ers and then coach Billy Walsh's famous West Coast Offence (Oriard, 2010: 95–139). Since then, broadcasters' use of video telestration has significantly contributed to the evolution of television production, with the inclusion of virtual graphics on a playing pitch now common place in any sports broadcasts (Pennington, 2014). Subsequently, the technology has driven enhancements such as virtual offside lines in soccer, as well as the dynamic line indicating world records during swimming and athletic events, all of which enrich viewer experience (Galily, 2014).

In recent years, the use of telestration has become regularly used in the broadcast of sports such as soccer, basketball, rugby union, netball, tennis, golf, and many others. The growing appetite of television audiences for tactically informed commentaries combined with the use of statistics and visualisation has seen the emergence of sportscasters that are analysing matches in greater analytical detail (Fele and Campagnolo, 2021). TV formats such as Sky's Monday Night Football (MNF) and TNT (formerly BT) Sport's Rugby Night have introduced specialist broadcast analysts who are tasked with delivering seamless tactical insight pre- and post-match, often incorporating the use of visual graphics. The success of telestration in a broadcast setting has led to the adoption of the technology in elite sport, particularly football (Bradley, 2020).

DOI: 10.4324/9781003375463-7

Video telestration provides an extension to traditional video analysis, which has been widely accepted to aid the recall of match events (Franks and Miller, 1986; Laird and Waters, 2008) and enhance the provision of feedback within the coaching process (Drust, 2010; Groom and Cushion, 2005; Nelson and Groom, 2012). Coaches and performance analysts now have opportunities to visualise the presentation of tactical, technical and physical performance parameters using integrated video and data (Bradley, 2020) and visually stimulating graphics (Fischer et al., 2019). Although several studies have explored the perceptions of performance analysis from the viewpoint of coaches, players and performance analysts (Butterworth et al., 2012; Francis and Jones, 2014; Nicholls et al., 2018; Wright et al., 2012), the evaluation of specific technological aids is less prevalent.

Outside of sport, telestration has been used in medical training to supplement verbal instruction, with its use leading to a reduction in overall training time required (Budrionis et al., 2013). The ability to annotate over video (Bogen et al., 2019) has been suggested to enhance the communication of information and reduce ambiguity and misunderstandings in verbal descriptions (Laborde et al., 2017). In a study by Budrionis et al. (2015), eight students participated in a randomised control trial that compared verbal and annotation-supplemented guidance from a remote mentor (e.g. telementoring). They found that telestration-supplemented guidance was quicker and led to a 33% decrease in training time. As well as this, most participants viewed the use of telestration positively (Budrionis et al., 2015). Despite the impact telestration has had in broadcast media and its potential in medical training, there have only been a small number of studies assessing the use and efficacy of video telestration technology within coaching and analysis environments.

Research into video telestration in sport

One of the first research studies to evaluate the use and application of telestration in sport was conducted by Jones et al. (2020). Using questionnaires, the study surveyed 58 professional coaches, players and performance analysts working in elite football clubs worldwide. The study confirmed the widespread use of video telestration in football environments and reported that a significant majority (93%) of respondents considered telestration "essential – very important" in everyday practice. Telestration was found to be used most frequently in preparation for matches, with 87% of respondents indicating that telestrated clips were produced for pre-match meetings and 85% of respondents reported viewing edited clips of opposition teams. Considering elite soccer teams have busy playing schedules and often play matches every two to three days (Dellal et al., 2015), the evidence supports the idea that tailored telestration video sequences can aid coaches and players prepare for competition against forthcoming opposition. Also, placing emphasis on the opposition is not surprising when opposition effect has been recognised as significantly influencing team and individual performance at a behavioural level

(McGarry and Franks, 2004). Only 50% of respondents reported telestration information informed the introduction and development of alterations in individual playing and tactical style. When evaluating the influence on individual player development, 42% of respondents indicated that telestration was 'fairly' influential. These percentages appear to be low considering that the overarching application of video analysis is to provide coaches with opportunities to analyse and create more sophisticated systems of play and aid the development of players tactical understanding (Cuevas et al., 2020). Of the analysts surveyed, 51% responded that telestration tools "aided retention" of information. However, with only anecdotal viewpoints and no empirical evidence in football, the researchers acknowledged the need to explore this in future research. Overall, the study by Jones et al. (2020) provides valuable insights into the prevalence and significance of video telestration in professional football, particularly in its support of opposition analysis.

Using a randomised control trial, Smith et al. (2022) measured the effectiveness of video telestration in memory recall of information of 14 professional soccer players. Half of the participants were randomly assigned to an experimental group with the other half forming a control group. The experimental group viewed telestrated video sequences, whereas the control group viewed non-telestrated video sequences. Participants viewed video sequences before completing a questionnaire 24 hours later. A 24-hour rest period followed, before participants repeated the process a total of five times over a period of 15 days. The study found that video telestration significantly enhanced memory recall and that participants who received telestrated video sequences recalled a greater amount of information (84.0% ± 3.7%) compared to those receiving non-telestrated video sequences (52.6% ± 5.4%). This indicates that telestration can improve memory recall of tactical information relating to possession, chance creation and set pieces by more than 30%. Interestingly, the recall of information relating to set pieces increased the most with telestrated (86.7%), compared to non-telestrated (48.0%) video sequences. Considering the importance of set pieces in elite soccer, telestration provides opportunities to support tactical improvement and inform teams' development of training (Leite, 2020). The authors acknowledged that increased levels of recall when using telestration could be attributed to (1) player familiarity with footage and opposition teams and (2) the number of graphics used on the video sequences. In summary, the study by Smith et al. (2022) is a valuable extension to the work by Jones et al. (2020) as it provides evidence that telestration does aid the retention of information in professional soccer players.

A further recommendation by Smith et al. (2022) was a need to evaluate the use of telestration with younger athletes. Røsseland (2018) undertook a study that evaluated the use of a single video telestration session (30 minutes in total) with 20 elite under-15 and under-16 football players from a Category 1 Norwegian Premier Division Academy. Like Smith et al.'s (2022) study, Røsseland (2018) used a randomised control trial but with ten participants in the control group (no-telestration) and ten in the video telestration group. All participants answered the same perceptual-cognitive skills questionnaire on three occasions, pre-, immediately post-session and seven days post-session. The questions relating to pattern recognition required participants to provide information on the 'identified' team's formation when out of position in the early phases of the opposition's build up play. Postural cue questions required players to identify which player would receive the ball from the player in possession. As there was no validated questionnaire to measure perceptual-cognitive skills, the questions were developed with the club's academy manager and utilised the framework developed by North et al. (2011) which looked at another cognitive skill (anticipation).

The results found that telestration significantly supported the participants' ability to recognise team formations (i.e. pattern recognition); however, the information was not retained over the seven-day measurement period. In comparison, immediately after the session, the telestration group were able to recall significantly more information compared to those who had video sequences without telestration. This finding supports the idea that telestration may be helpful in short term planning (e.g. for matches against forthcoming opposition), which was identified previously as a core use of telestration in elite soccer (Jones et al., 2020). Interestingly, both telestrated and non-telestrated video sequences improved postural cue usage (i.e., action being undertaken by the player with the ball), including retention over the seven-day measurement. This result provides evidence one video (training) session alone regardless of the presence of telestration can contribute to the development of such an important skill (Smeeton et al., 2018). Nevertheless, further evidence and the evaluation of longer-term exposure to telestration is required. Røsseland's (2018) use of video (training) and telestration supports an ecological approach that considers the interaction between performer, their environment and required tasks (Araujo et al., 2006). As such the methodological approach differs to perceptual training methods, where concern has been raised about how improvements observed in controlled laboratory settings can translate to performance (North and Williams, 2019). Although Rosseland's (2018) study is only based on one video (training) session, the questionnaire lacked validity and the transfer effects to match play require longitudinal consideration, it provides some interesting results regarding the use of video (training) and telestration to evaluate postural cues and pattern recognition. Moreover, the study draws attention to the use of video telestration technology and its potential to contribute to an emerging scientific research area within performance analysis.

Telestration software and features

Whilst there is some evidence to support the use and effectiveness of telestration in soccer (Jones et al., 2020; Røsseland, 2018; Smith et al., 2022), effective use of appropriate graphics in the correct context is vitally important when creating video sequences (Bradley, 2020). This should be a consideration when using telestration software in a coaching and analysis setting. Telestration tools are now provided within some commercial video analysis packages, such as Hudl

Studio (Hudl, Lincoln, NE), Play (Metrica Sports, Amsterdam, Netherlands), KlipDraw Animate (Nacsport, Gran Canaria, Spain), Dartfish Pro (Dartfish, Fribourg, Switzerland), Focus (Catapult Sports, Melbourne, Australia), and are also available in specialist packages, such as Tactic Pro (RT Software, London, UK), Coach Paint (ChyronHego, Melville, NY), Vizrt (Viz Libero, Bergen, Norway) and Piero (Ross Video, Ottawa, Canada) to post-process video clips. Common telestration graphics within software packages include freehand lines, directional arrows, player cursors (e.g. individual or linked with lines), player trails (e.g. lines behind player), player highlights (e.g. light shafts and magnifier), pitch zones/regions (e.g. circles and rectangles) and text graphics (e.g. titles and player tags). More advanced graphics include 3D arrows and graphics with measurement capabilities, such as for distance and speed.

Although research into video telestration in sport has placed an emphasis on football, this chapter will also consider use within team sports more broadly. The next section will focus on describing how to use the specialist telestration software Tactic Pro and use other examples from specialist packages and telestration tools available in commercial packages where appropriate. The following technical aspects of video telestration will be covered as subsections (1) chroma key, calibration and motion (camera) tracking and (2) manual key framing and player detection.

Chroma keyer, calibration and motion (camera) tracking

Prior to the augmentation of a video with graphics, the user must identify a relevant video sequence to highlight players and action of interest. The next process is to apply the chroma keyer. Using soccer as an example, this is achieved by using the chroma keyer to detect a dominant colour (i.e. green of playing pitch). Once set, this allows graphics to be placed above the pitch and appear behind a player. This is an example of simple image processing which allows graphics to appear drawn on the ground and not on top of players or other objects, adding the element of realism that they are "painted" on the pitch (Thomas et al., 2017). There are two common ways to detect the chroma keyer in packages, the first is with automatic chroma keyer detection and the second is where the user manually applies the key using a picker tool (Figure 7.1). A frequent problem with video clips from soccer stadia are shadows on the pitch, in this instance a combination of automatic and manual keying may be required.

A vital process that must be undertaken when working with telestration software is camera calibration, which allows users to render graphics to a pitch, so they appear 'tied-to-pitch' (Thomas et al., 2017). Calibration requires the user to overlay a 3D model on the pitch surface (Figure 7.2). This is achieved by using prominent line markers and defined pitch positions such as the middle and extremities of a pitch, commonly referred to as line-based trackers (Thomas, 2007). Calibration also enables users to use graphics with measurement capabilities (e.g. distance tools and player physical distance tracking). Some packages require the user to run a camera track (Tactic Pro) or enable motion tracking (Coach Paint) in the graphic tool properties.

Many software packages now have the capability to run automatic chroma keying and camera calibration. Though these processes expedite the preparation of video sequences, the success of these automated processes will be influenced by the quality of the original video, angle and perspective being used and sport. Users should ensure that they are familiar with the steps required to prepare a video before applying any graphics.

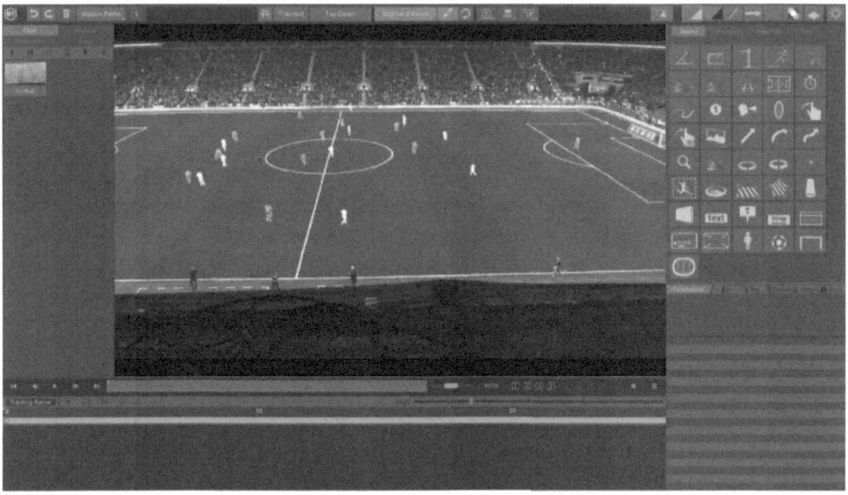

Figure 7.1 Chroma keyer: in the example, the Chroma keyer has been set manually using the "segment" keyer to show the detection of the dominant colour (e.g., Pitch).

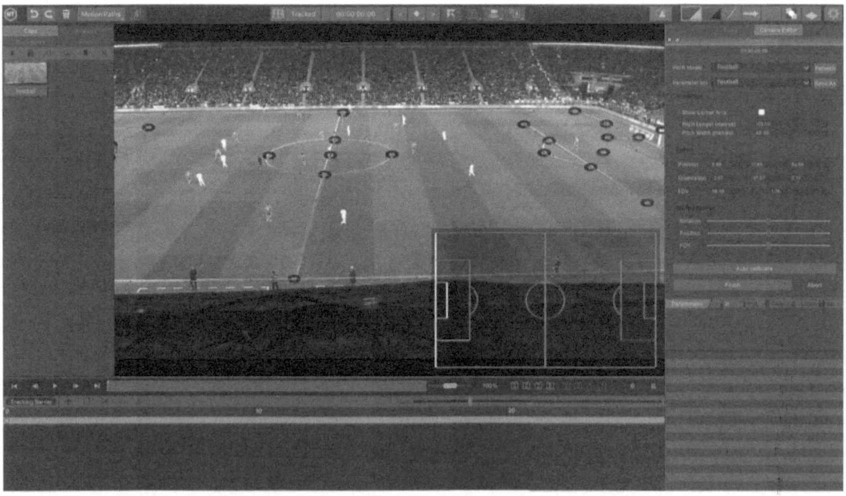

Figure 7.2 Pitch Calibration: the 3D pitch model can be changed according to sport (e.g., Football, Rugby, Gaelic Football) and parameters such as pitch length and width can be adjusted if the size of pitch is known.

Manual key framing and player detection

To track an object (i.e. a player) with a moving graphic, a user must manually follow the player as the video progresses, dragging and dropping the graphic for a specified amount of time creates a key frame pathway (Figure 7.3). Single or multiple graphics can be added to the key frame path of the player and the user can set "in" and "out" points for the graphics. Key frames can also be adjusted or deleted if necessarily. Specialist packages, such as Tactic and Coach Paint, have automatic player detection (e.g. tracking), a process that utilises computer vision and Artificial Intelligence (AI) technology to track a single player or all players in a video sequence with bounding boxes (e.g. Rahimian and Toka, 2022). As a result of this process, the software creates a key frame pathway (Figure 7.4). An advantage of automatic tracking is the time it saves the user as it significantly reduces the requirement to manually enter key frames for players when using graphics. This is particularly helpful when a user needs to add a graphic to highlight the movement of a single player or group of players (e.g. team formations) for a period of a video sequence. Tracking within Hudl Studio is different to Tactic and Coach Paint; rather than tracking all players, the system can follow an object (such as a player disc) automatically.

Automatic player detection and the AI models in telestration software are not without fault, for example, bounding boxes and key frame paths can be lost or change to follow a different player when players cross in front and behind of each other in a video sequence. When this happens, users are required to correct the errors manually by reconnecting or adding new key frame paths. Undoubtedly with more training and data, AI models will improve over time. Users should utilise player detection and automated tracking to expedite processes. However, a fundamental principle of telestration is manual key framing graphics, therefore users should endeavour to develop this core skill.

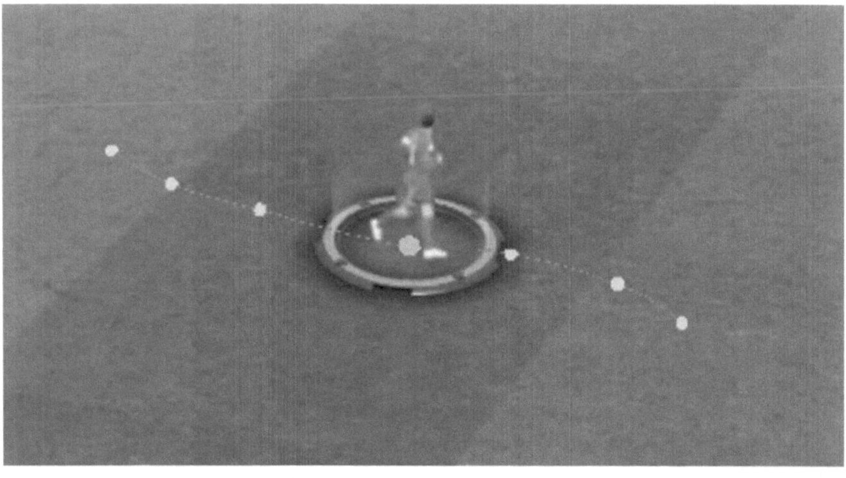

Figure 7.3 Manual Keyframing: by dragging and dropping a graphic (e.g., 3D Cursor) for a specified amount of time, the user creates a keyframe pathway. Graphic inpoint and output can easily be set using keyboard shortcuts.

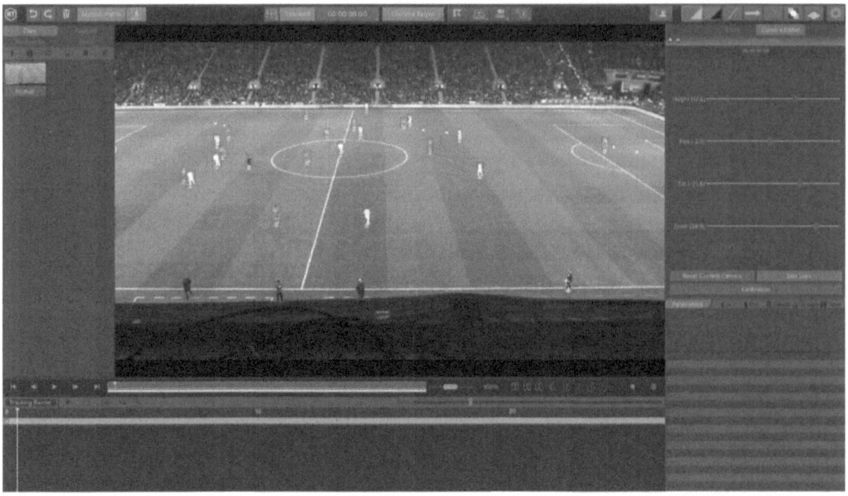

Figure 7.4 Player Detection: a bounding box is added around each player and motion (keyframe) paths are added. If a graphic (e.g., 3D cursor) is added to a player, it will automatically follow the player until an outpoint is set. This alleviates the need to manually track the player.

Applying graphics

This section uses three examples to illustrate the processes of telestration. These examples are for counterattacks in soccer, defensive pressure in field hockey and tactical decision making in rugby union.

Example 1. Visualising a counterattack in soccer

Figure 7.5a shows the initial phase of a soccer counterattack. The initial points of interest are the player on the ball (Davies), who initiates the counterattack and the movement of the attacking player, who is dropping deep into the space between the opposition's defence and midfield, dragging the defending team's central defender out of position. In Figure 7.5b, the two wide players have been highlighted with a linked cursor (and distance measure). This is to highlight the width both players are maintaining on the pitch. This combination of technical and tactical information is helpful to add context to the game situation. A cursor with a trail has been used to continually track the forward run of the player (Davies). In Figure 7.5c, a pitch zone graphic has been added alongside two directional arrows; the first directional arrow indicates the potential continuation of the attacking player's forward run and the second is highlighting the impact this has had on the defending team's central defender, who has chosen to engage with the developing attacking situation (as a consequence of being drawn out of position earlier in the sequence). In Figure 7.5d, the counterattack has progressed to a 4–3 overload in favour of the attacking team. The four attacking players are identified with player titles and the opposition's defensive structure has been highlighted with a linked cursor. A pitch zone (region graphic) and directional arrow have been included to highlight the free space that the right-sided winger (Bale) can move into as play evolves.

The analysis of counter attacks is highly beneficial for both attacking and defending teams, as the information can inform both pre and most match

(a)

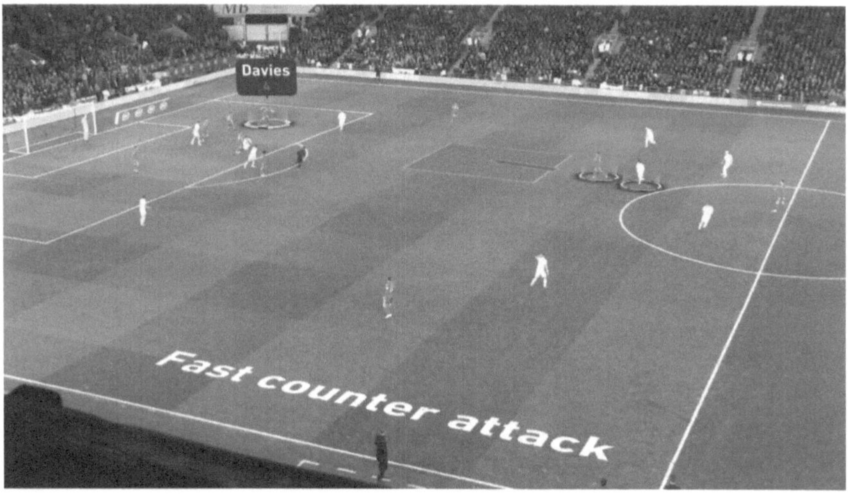

(b)

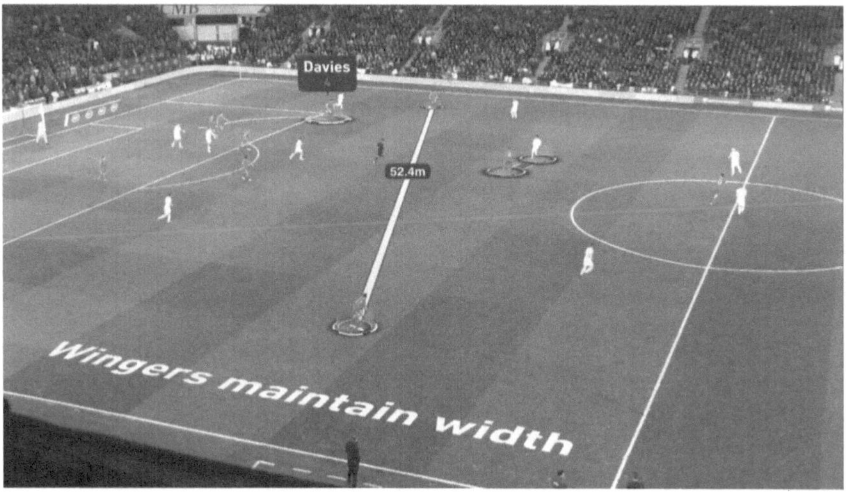

Figure 7.5 (a) Davies (cursor and player tag) initiating counterattack and teammate moving towards centre of pitch (region tool, directional arrow and cursor). (b) Forward run of Davies tracked (cursor with trail), position of wingers highlighted (linked cursor and distance) and attacking player and defender connected (linked cursor). *(Continued)*

(c)

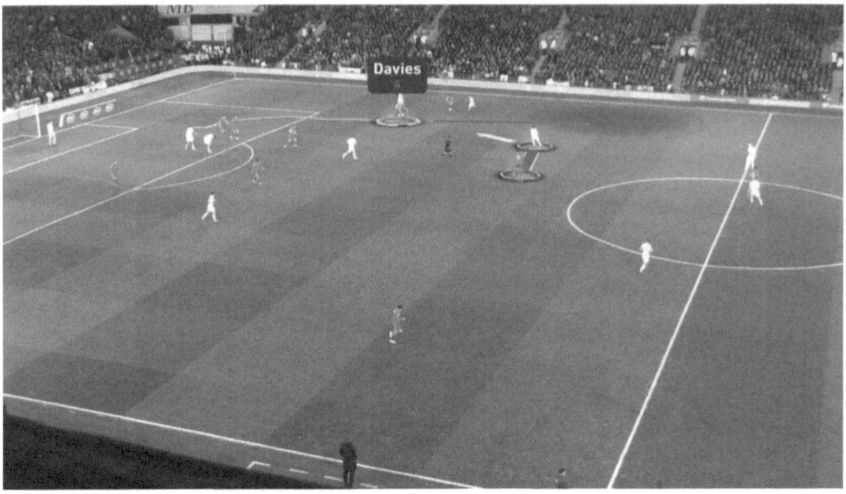

(d)

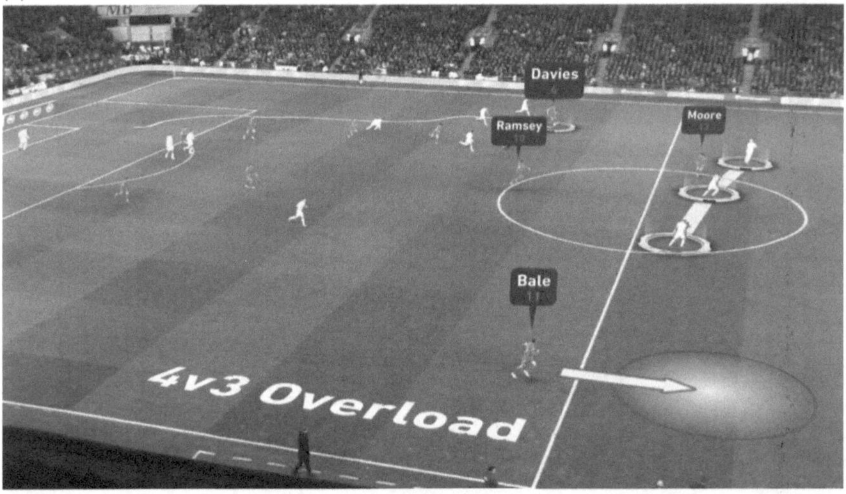

Figure 7.5 (Continued) (c) Potential player movements (directional arrows) towards highlighted areas (region tool). (d) Counterattack evolved into 4–3 attacking situation. Attacking players identified (player tags) and opposition defensive structure highlighted (linked cursor).

reviews. Through the visualisation of the offensive possession in the current example, it is possible to establish an understanding of team tendencies, such as the first action after recovering the ball (e.g. dribble or pass) and areas of the pitch (e.g. central or wide areas) teams develop attacking play from (Sarmento et al., 2014). It is noted that additional video evidence is needed to build a comprehensive understanding of teams' attacking tendencies. Additional graphics can also support the visualisation of physical performance parameters in soccer, and these include metrics such as distance covered (m) and the speed of player ($m.s^{-1}$) during phases of play (Bradley, 2020). Readers with a keen interest in the visualisation of data and video in soccer are encouraged to access The FIFA Football Language which is available open source on the FIFA Training Centre (FIFA, n.d.). There are a variety of resources and example telestrations that have been created to visualise different tactical aspects of play.

Example 2. Visualising defensive pressure in field hockey

Another sport that can benefit from the use of telestration is field hockey. Figure 7.6a shows a defensive team's diamond midfield (region tool) and front three players (linked cursor) in field hockey. The top forward has an additional graphic (lightshaft) to suggest the player has split the pitch and is forcing the player in possession to move to the left. The distance (7.8m) between the midfielder at the top of the diamond and the right-sided forward player is included to provide additional technical information. As the sequence progresses (Figure 7.6b), the team in possession takes the opportunity to play a penetrative pass through the forward and midfield line. Figure 7.6c shows the opposition player (cursor) has been able to receive the ball in a passing lane, turn, and then dribble forward under little pressure, before passing the ball to a teammate. The visualisation also includes the distance covered by the two defending players in their attempt to close the opposition player down. As an intermittent high intensity and dynamic sport where playing position (e.g. midfielder and forward) can

(a)

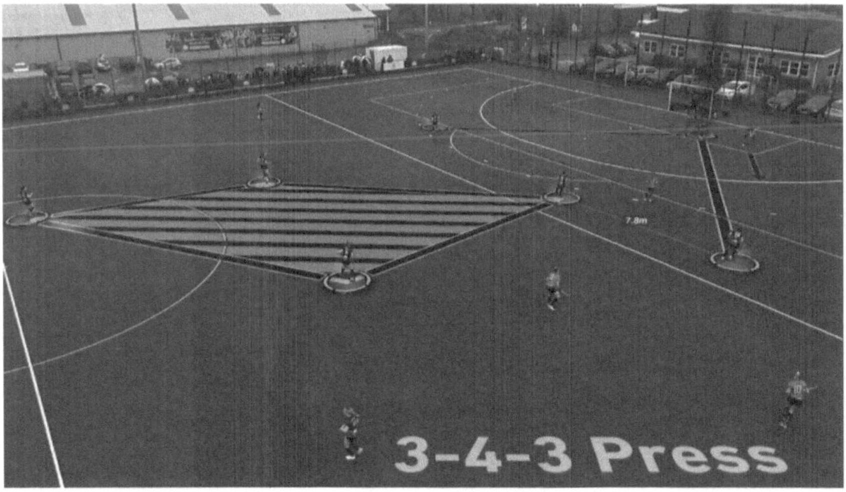

Figure 7.6 (a) Visualisation of defensive structure with region, cursors and directional arrows. *(Continued)*

(b)

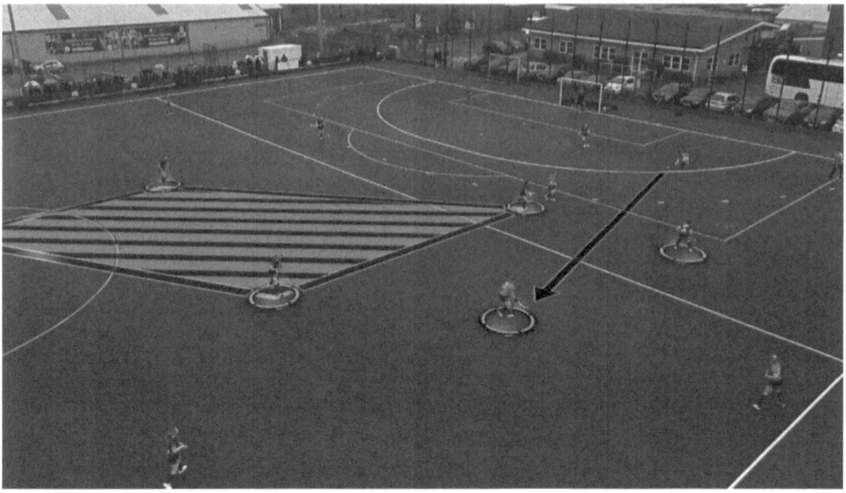

(c)

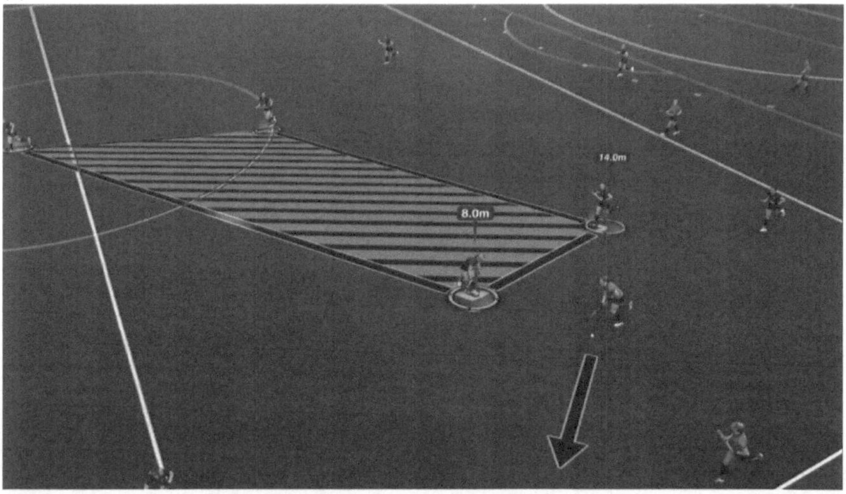

Figure 7.6 (Continued) (b) Penetrative pass between midfield and forward line. (c) Physical performance parameters to add contextual information.

significantly impact physical output (Jennings, 2012). The inclusion of physical performance parameters, such as distance covered by the players before applying a defensive action, can help add further context to the technical-tactical demands of game play. In the current example, the opposition team have demonstrated an ability to move the ball quickly and exploit the defensive structure of the opposition (Cunniffe et al., 2022). The use of graphics and information could inform the defending team's post-match review about where they may need to make adjustments to prevent penetrative passes.

Example 3. Evaluating tactical decision making in rugby union

Figure 7.7a shows an attacking phase of play in rugby union. The focus in this clip is the evaluation of decision making by the attacking player (fly half/ Number 10), who has the ball in hand and is highlighted with a cursor and lightshaft in the centre of the pitch. The defending fullback for the opposition team is also highlighted with a cursor and a directional arrow to indicate intended defensive movement. The fly half has four "potential" options highlighted with arrows and numbers (1–4); the first is a flat pass to the next player in the backline (1). Other options include a "miss" pass option to players in position 2 (centre), 3 (fullback) or 4 (winger). However, the potential pass to the player in position 4 (winger) appears to be a risky option with the opposition player (winger) on the outside look to fold in and make a tackle. Attacking player 4 (winger) does, however, have a raised arm and is signalling to the attacking number 10 (Figure 7.7b). The use of the magnifier tool in this instance is beneficial to draw attention to a specific action taking place in the video sequence. In Figure 7.7c, the area behind the defensive line (region graphic) is highlighted and a 3D arrow has been added to indicate the option of a kick in behind the defensive line for the attacker. Advanced tools such as 3D arrows (to indicate flight of the ball) combined with other graphics offer increased insight not possible with traditional video analysis (Bradley, 2020).

Coaches have widely reported the use of post-game video analysis as an approach to analysis and for improving player decision making (Morgan et al., 2020; O'Connor and Larkin, 2015). The example visualises "various" options available to the player and can support reflection on a key decision-making moment from a match. The graphics highlight the evolving technical and

(a)

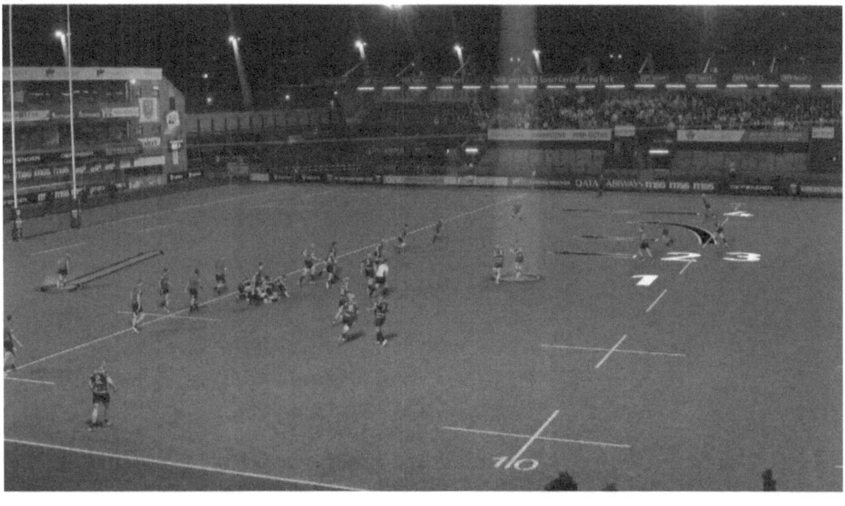

Figure 7.7 (a) Initial phase of play developing outside of the opposition 22. The number 10 (fly half) is highlighted (spotlight) as well as the four attacking players/options (directional arrows and numbers). *(Continued)*

(b)

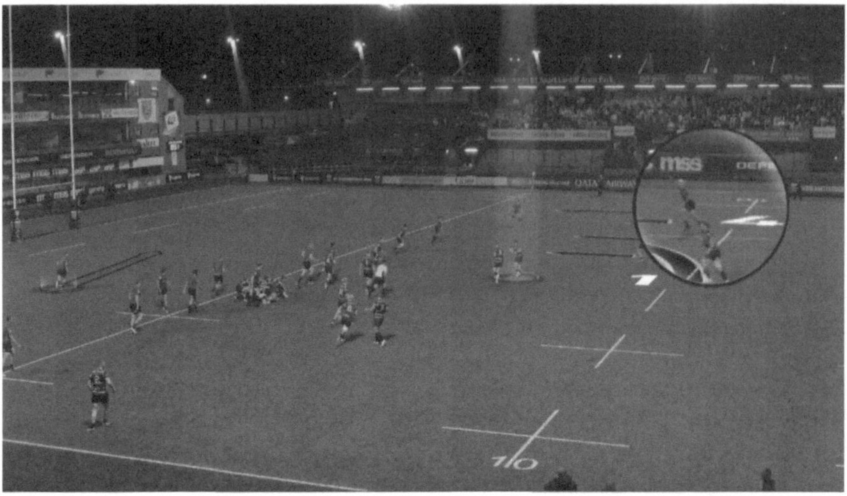

(c)

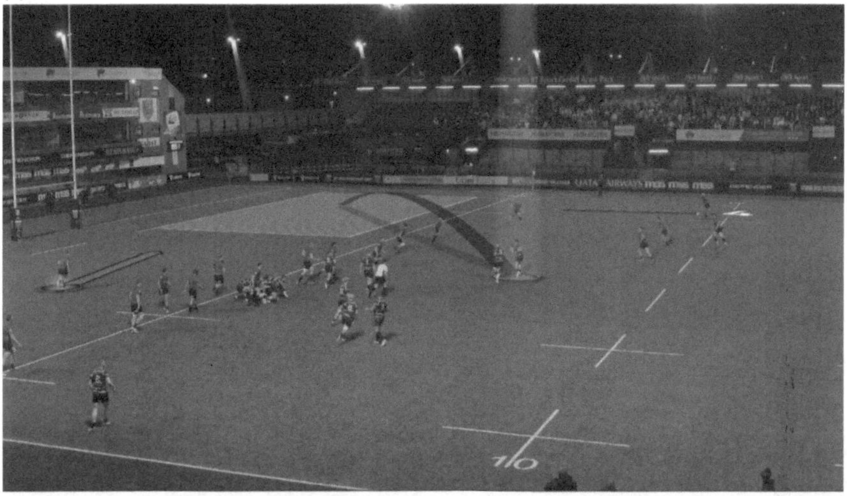

Figure 7.7 (Continued) (b) Magnifier tool showing the raised hand (subtle action) of the winger. The rest of the image is masked/greyed out, drawing attention to the circle in the top right corner. (c) A region graphic has been used to highlight the space behind the defensive line and a 3D arrow has been added to indicate the kicking option and trajectory required for a kick in behind the defensive line.

tactical picture of the game (phase of play) and factors that may influence the player's decision making, such as the situation and the location of teammates and the opposition (O'Connor and Larkin, 2015). Furthermore, when assessing decision making, there is a need to separate the "decision made" and the "execution" of the skill (Lorains et al., 2013). In the current example, the fly half could make the (best) decision, which is to kick in behind the defence, but execute the kick poorly. Alternatively, a flat pass to the next attacking player could be executed perfectly, but in the context of the play, this may be deemed the 2nd best option. Therefore, the use of graphics should support discussion(s) between the player, coach and other teammates to evaluate the decision-making situation. Building on this, the next section in this chapter will explore the presentation and feedback capabilities of telestration and opportunities for interaction during analysis and feedback sessions.

Presentation and feedback

Whilst the last sections focused on the doing of telestration of work, the following section will discuss how users can share telestration outputs with coaches and players. Should users wish to share video sequences (such as those in the previous section), they can export single or multiple videos from telestration packages to be integrated into commercial video analysis packages or other presentation programs (e.g. Microsoft PowerPoint or iWork Keynote). Alternatively, specialist packages such as Tactic Pro and Coach Paint also have integrated presentation modes which allow users to change the software's interface and present via touchscreen monitors and tablet devices. These features provide coaches, analysts and players with intuitive ways to engage in video-based feedback and communication. In touchscreen mode, users can play, pause and control the playback speed of video clips whilst adding real-time graphics at various intervals to illustrate key points, embracing the origins of the broadcast 'telestrator' discussed earlier in this chapter. The software's graphical user interface (GUI) can be customised to include a set number and type of graphics, both of which depend on the purpose of the analysis and preference of the user. Using the example in Figure 7.8, this could commonly include free hand lines, directional arrows, player cursors (e.g. individual or linked with lines), player highlights (e.g. light shafts/magnifier) and region zones (e.g. circles and rectangles).

Prior to working with a clip in the presentation mode, users should still follow the steps of identifying a relevant clip, chroma keying and calibration outlined earlier in this chapter. Clips can be added to the presentation mode 'clean' (i.e. without graphics), in this instance the user controls video playback, and at each pause can added graphics. When the video resumes graphics can be made to disappear from screen using a 'clear on play' function. Alternatively, a user may wish to combine this with a telestrated video sequence and use touchscreen capability to add additional graphics. An example of this may be the desire to track the movement of a single player or unit of players. Therefore, it is advisable that these graphics are already added to the clip.

An extension to working with a touchscreen is tablet controls, a feature available within both Tactic Pro and Coach Paint. The feature works by connecting a laptop running the telestration software and a tablet to the same

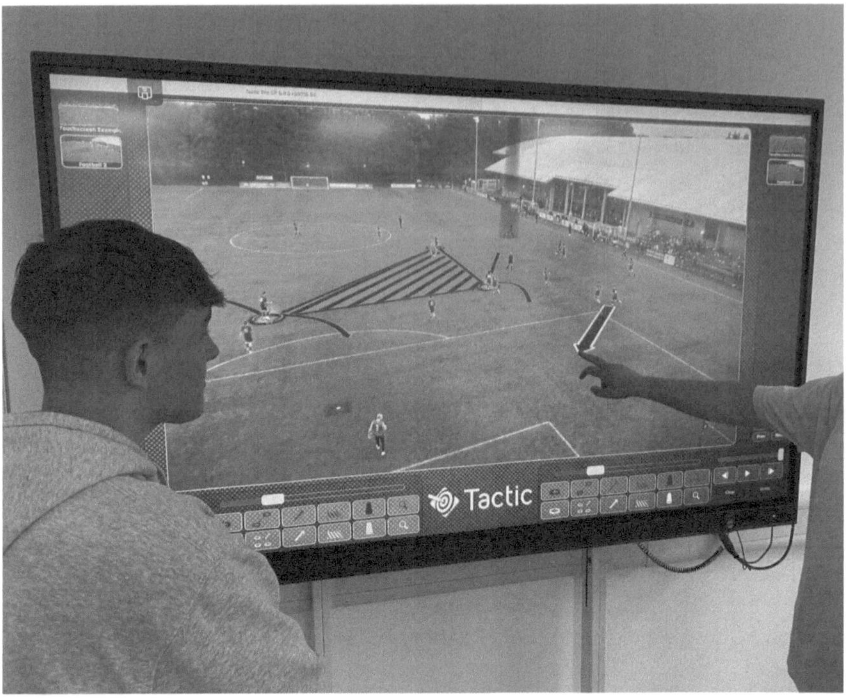

Figure 7.8 Use of touchscreen by player during team meeting.

network, with the control panel accessible by inputting an Internet Protocol (IP) address into a web browser on the tablet. Once connected, users can draw graphics in real-time on the tablet (Figure 7.9), and if the laptop system is connected to a project, screen graphics will appear simultaneously. The tactile nature of touchscreens and tablets provides opportunities for analysts, coaches and players to engage in communication and the exchange of ideas (i.e. interaction) during video-based coaching and analysis sessions.

Pedagogical use of video telestration

Video analysis commonly provides coaches with the opportunity to prepare for matches (e.g. opposition analysis) and post-match, evaluate strengths and weaknesses of team and individual performance (Wright et al., 2014). In this regard, utilising video sequences with accompanying verbal feedback has been recognised as a beneficial approach to facilitating player learning and encouraging reflection on performance (Groom and Cushion, 2005; Groom et al., 2011). Although the research by Smith et al. (2022) discussed earlier in this chapter highlighted the influence telestration had on players' ability to recall information and suggested learning occurred, the links between video telestration technology and learning require further evidence. Approaches to

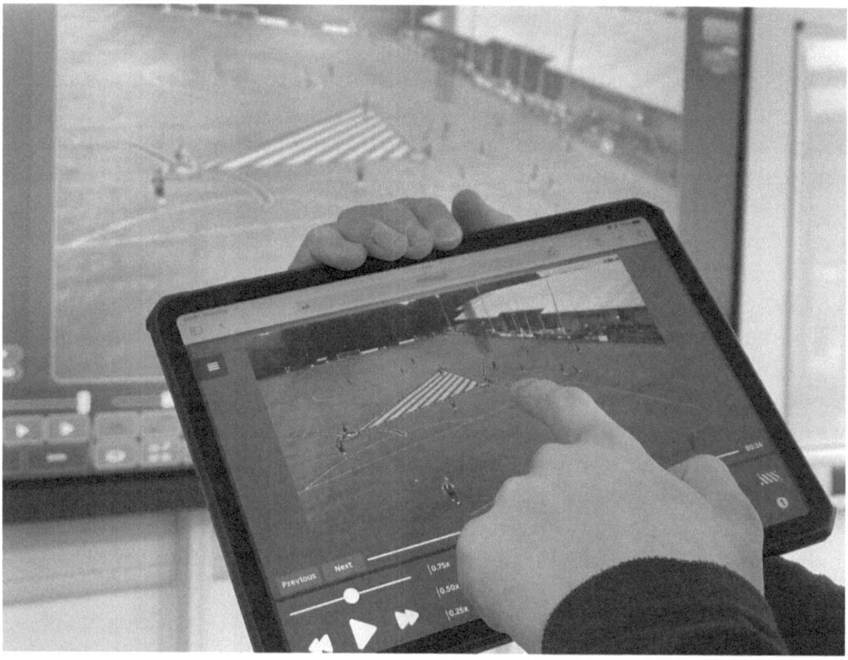

Figure 7.9 Tablet Control in RT Tactic.

the delivery of video-based feedback can vary, though one popular method is via audio-visual (AV) technology in a large setting, which implies a video feedback session has similarities to a classroom setting (Mason et al., 2021). However, despite the widespread use and benefits of video feedback, there has been limited research into the delivery methods (including telestration) used by coaches and the pedagogy (i.e. teaching and learning) of video analysis with coaches and athletes (Groom and Nelson, 2013). Furthermore, with evidence to suggest that the learning dynamics of coaches and players are intricate, and the influence of video analysis on player learning and overall team tactical understanding is not a simple or direct process (Brümmer, 2019). This challenges traditional approaches that coaches sharing video alone leads to individual learning and reflection (Carling et al., 2005).

When delivering video feedback sessions, activities that promote learners (players) to actively participate in the process (e.g. engage in meaningful discussion) can lead to increased learning opportunities (Wright et al., 2016). An example of this is the study by Thomas and Edwards (2022) who applied an innovative use of Piotr Galperin's (six) teaching and learning framework and video (analysis) telestration to develop pedagogical practice and soccer players' tactical understanding. For more information on Galperin's pedagogical framework, refer to Engeness and Lund (2020). Using an action research design, Thomas and Edwards's study took place over a five-month period at a semi-professional soccer club, with data collected using a combination of video analysis focus groups and semi-structured interviews. Guided by the learning framework, participants had opportunities to discuss tactical options and use telestration technology to add graphics in real-time onto video clips. All players in the study acknowledged the value interacting with the technology (e.g. telestration) had on developing their tactical understanding and enjoyed having the opportunity to critically discuss each other's decisions. This work demonstrates that active participation, social interaction and the use of telestration technology can lead to a meaningful learning experience and provides evidence of the development of collective tactical understanding.

Despite the study's in-depth findings, Thomas and Edwards's acknowledged two limitations in their qualitative methodology. The first limitation draws attention to the study taking place within one football club and the use of an interpretive paradigm, suggesting researchers may choose to use alternative paradigms (e.g., positivism) and different methodologies to explore the research topic. The second limitation is the retrospective nature of the data collection and accounts from coaches' and players. Future telestration (video analysis) research should consider the transfer of learning from the 'interactive classroom' to the playing pitch. This could potential be achieved through first-hand observation of live training sessions and/or implementation of telestration (video) interventions in a live training session. Furthermore, the effect on performance-related variables (e.g., technical effectiveness) and performance should also be considered. This is yet to be considered by research into video telestration in sport.

The significance of the research by Thomas and Edwards (2022) is that it considers the development of collective tactical understanding and contributes to developing an understanding of how technology, such as telestration, is used at the technology-coach-player-learning interface. There are other examples of qualitative research into the complexities surrounding the delivery of video feedback (e.g. Groom et al., 2012; Magill et al., 2017; Nelson et al., 2014; Raya-Castellano, 2020). However, due to the fact many explore various other facets of video analysis delivery, not the specific use of telestration technology, these are not covered in this chapter. Readers interested in qualitative research within this area should review these papers and continue to the next chapter that discusses the communication of feedback within sport performance analysis.

Telestration benefits, challenges and future considerations

Though this chapter identifies benefits to the use of telestration, such as its role in helping teams preview opposition, recall important information and engage players within learning, there are still a series of associated challenges. These include significant financial costs to acquire telestration software, the expertise required to conduct telestration and time implications to its use

(Jones et al., 2020). More expensive packages are those that have been developed in broadcast settings but have now cascaded down into elite sporting environments. The advantages of specialist telestration packages include an increased variety of graphics, additional features (e.g. integration of external player tracking data sources) and capability to run in presentation modes. However, the growth of telestration has driven many commercial video analysis software providers to integrate telestration tools into their software packages, which in turn has made telestration more accessible to all levels of sports, not just elite teams and organisations.

With continual automation of technology such as video capture and detection of match events, there is less requirement for analysts to undertake time consuming tasks such as "filming" and "manual data entry". In principle, this should afford analysts more time to engage in the "analysis and contextualisation of performance". This is particularly pertinent when it is widely accepted that coaches and players hold a preference for video-based feedback (Bradley, 2020; Wright et al., 2014). Therefore, video telestration with its ability to contribute to the creation of stimulating learning resources and activities for coaches and players will undoubtedly continue to grow. Job adverts reinforce widespread use, with many stipulating applied analysts to have experience in the use of video telestration (visualisation) software. As an important technical competency, aspiring and current analysts should endeavour to develop their knowledge and understanding in effective use (e.g. pedagogical and time efficiencies). This could be developed during a programme of study (e.g. undergraduate or postgraduate degrees), work placement or formal training from software providers. In fast-paced high-performance environments where the analyst is often the human at the interface between technology-video-data, possessing the abilities to communicate effectively (Robertson, 2020) and transfer information into insight quickly and without overload is important (Bradley, 2020).

Conclusions

Current research supports the idea that telestration has the potential to enhance video-based feedback and communication between coaches, players and analysts. More specifically, teams' preparation for matches (e.g. opposition analysis), ability to accurately recall essential information on performance and improve tactical knowledge and understanding can all be enhanced. In addition, the use of advanced graphics and associated metrics can help contextualise tactical, technical and physical information sources within telestrated video sequences. This is extremely helpful and can support the creation of tailored telestrated video sequences to engage players and coaches in feedback processes, extending traditional video analysis practices. However, there is no standardised approach to using graphics within video sequences. Therefore, the authors acknowledge there are many ways to apply graphics and the examples provided throughout this chapter are for example purposes. To date, video telestration research in sport has focused on its use in soccer (predominantly with senior players). Therefore, it would be beneficial to expand research into different demographics (e.g. age and gender) and different sports (e.g. team and individual). For example, there is also a need for further research into the pedagogical use of video telestration (e.g. technology) and how it contributes to active participation and social interaction during the delivery and discussion of video-based feedback in coaching and analysis. Additionally, further understanding of the transferability of learning from (classroom) to on-pitch and the effect on performance-related variables and performance would also be welcomed within future research.

8 Communicating feedback

Introduction

The work and role of a performance analyst does not stop at the conclusion of a sporting performance. In fact, the analysis of a performance using a pre-designed and tested template is only the beginning (input phase), with the throughput and output phases following in the cyclical process. This chapter will focus on the output phase of the analysis process. In this instance, data has been collected and analysed and key performance indicators have been generated which have associated video sequences (see Chapter 5). The role of the performance analyst now shifts to communicating the collected information to audiences in the best way to enhance learning within the given context. Knowing that the effective delivery of extrinsic feedback can complement intrinsic information (Maslovat and Franks, 2020), this chapter discusses presenting performance analysis results and includes tips for delivering feedback.

Role clarity and expectations

At the commencement of any new season or in a new position as a performance analyst, it is vitally important to check in with management teams away from training and match environments, to gain clarity on the analysts' roles and responsibilities. Traditionally, match day or training environments are exceptionally busy with each practitioner having their own duties prior to a practice session or performance commencing. Therefore, in order to have a conducive working environment and an opportunity to discuss performance analysis provision in detail, it would be advised to organise a time and place that suits all parties outside of these busy environments.

Regardless of the analyst's level of experience, their time at the organisation or the coaches' level of buy-in into performance analysis provision, this platform provides an opportunity to develop relationships, gain an understanding of shared language and in some cases an appreciation of working within a multidisciplinary team. This is an opportunity to raise how performance analysis can be used to support athletes, coaches and the wider team which may lead to collaborative opportunities. Naturally, these discussions will require performance analysts to draw on their interpersonal skills to

DOI: 10.4324/9781003375463-8

develop relationships and communicate effectively and, in some scenarios, the requirement of negotiating with individuals (Bateman and Jones, 2019). The quality of the coach-analyst relationship is vital; so important that it sees coaches recruit performance analysts who they have previously worked with (Huggan et al., 2015). These strong professional working relationships are critical to the effective delivery of performance analysis provision (Martin et al., 2021) and time must be prioritised to establish these relationships.

In an attempt to contextualise factors raised above, a scenario of a performance analyst starting a new role has been developed below:

> *My first week as a performance analyst! An exciting time but I was also so nervous. It felt a little unconformable not knowing exactly what I was supposed to be doing or where anything was, but it did get better as the week went on. I'm already looking forward to next week. Everyone seems nice, so far; I can't remember all of their names yet but that'll come, I'm sure. On Tuesday, I saw the manager in the corridor quickly, he looked busy and pretty flustered but it was just before training. It was nice though because we met properly on Wednesday at the coffee shop. He seems friendly and we talked about sport and other things too, which was nice. I didn't realise how new he was to this coaching role and I'm the first performance analyst he's worked with. We spoke generally about what he and the team want, but I do need to go back to him with ideas on sharing operational definitions. He has mentioned that the assistant coach isn't too keen on performance analysis though, which might be a handful. He didn't go into too much detail, but it seems he may have had a bad experience as a player. Apparently, he's happy to receive some stats but he's not too keen on the video side of things.*

During role clarity conversations, it is also assumed that much of the discussion will align to the input phase of performance analysis, this concerning the data collection phase, confirmation of key performance indicators and the definition of their terms, e.g., defining of a positive tackle or the affirmation of the final third area. Yet, it is also important to explore the general expectations of performance analysis provision in all other environments, and this includes the expectancies within in a training environment and the expectations of analysis post-performance. This might include questions such as: How promptly post-performance is analysis expected? How will the data and video be shared? How will feedback be communicated and delivered? How would the coach like this to look? How will the analysis be used? How might we measure the effectiveness of delivery styles and information provided? So, while conversations on the input phase are important, it is equally important to have conversations regarding the output of provision. Feedback is an invaluable aspect impacting learning (Maslovat and Franks, 2020) yet to provide meaningful instruction and advice, a complete perspective of performance must be attained. With the work of Franks and Miller (1991) and later Laird and Waters (2008), the natural demand for performance analysis has elevated to ensure this record of performance is collected. It is through negotiations with coaches and athletes, that decisions can be made on how this information is communicated.

Coaching process models

The coaching process is thought of as a complex ongoing cycle of performance, analysis and feedback (Maslovat and Franks, 2020). Coaching models (Hughes and Franks, 2008; O'Donoghue and Mayes, 2013) indicate that this is conducted at both training and match environments (during and post-performance) and, in some cases, includes the analysis of opposition (Groom et al., 2011; Horne et al., 2013; Wright et al., 2014). Whilst many models recognise the processes involved in the collection of data and video, the use and delivery of video-based feedback are equally as important considerations (Groom & Nelson, 2013). This has seen the development of coaching process models based on the application of performance analysis in practice, which have attempted to acknowledge the actual delivery and communication of video feedback. In that regard, Groom et al. (2011) and O'Donoghue and Mayes (2013) developed models with greater consideration for athlete learning and reflection.

The use and application of analysis has similarities to the four key stages of action research; these are observing, reflecting, planning and acting. O'Donoghue and Mayes (2013) tailored this approach to performance analysis activities in the coaching process (Figure 8.1).

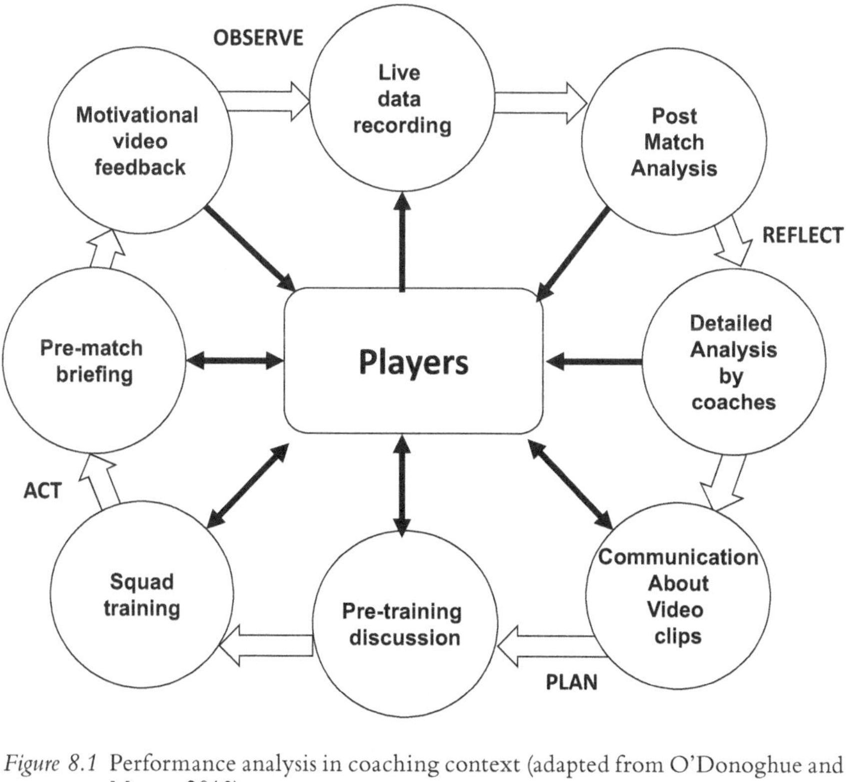

Figure 8.1 Performance analysis in coaching context (adapted from O'Donoghue and Mayes, 2013).

Similarly, Wright et al. (2014) proposed a model of stages, which also included observation and planning, as well as stages for analysis, interpreting and preparation. When comparing both models, a strength of O'Donoghue and Mayes (2013) is the incorporation of a reflection stage, which can be used to aid and facilitate athlete learning. Here, task details included performance analysts uploading and sharing video sequences to a password protected analysis site, for the squad to discuss and reflect on, prior to future training sessions. Most importantly, O'Donoghue and Mayes' (2013) athlete-centred approach encourages a two-way communication of sharing information back and forth between coaches and players, thus creating an equitable power balance between roles.

With the desire to understand video-analysis practices in applied coaching environments, Groom et al. (2011) developed a theoretical framework from a grounded theory research methodology. The study established how contextual factors such as social environment, coaching philosophy and recipient qualities influenced the delivery of video-based feedback (Figure 8.2). In light of these findings, it is evident that coaches' delivery of video-based feedback to support athlete learning is a complex process.

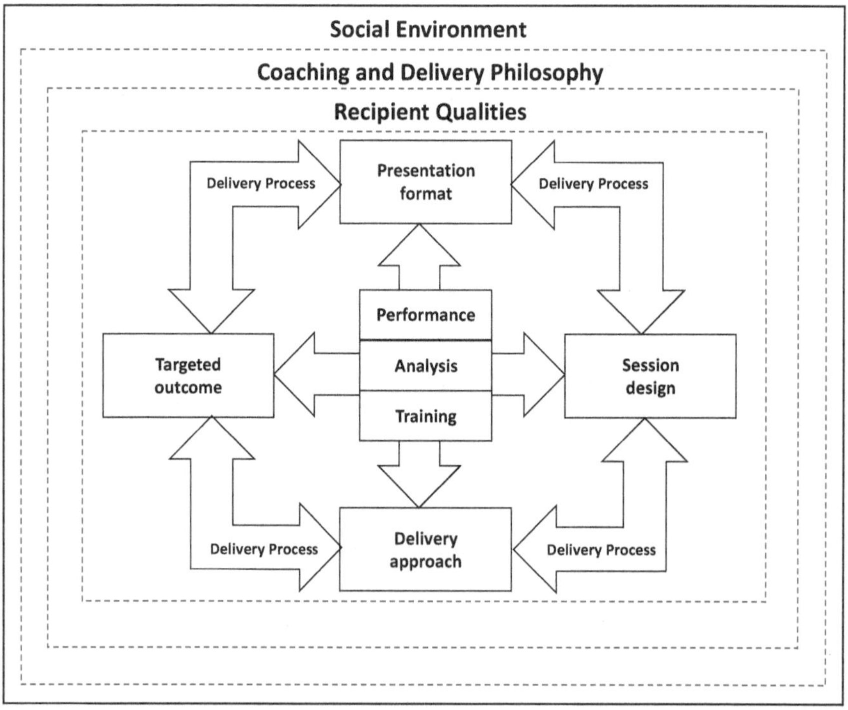

Figure 8.2 A grounded theory of the delivery of video-based performance analysis feedback (adapted from Groom et al., 2011).

The next section will discuss in more depth the contextual factors that influence the delivery of video-based analysis, these will include coach leadership style, delivery approaches, and presentation types.

Contextual Factors

Prior to communicating any feedback, Martin et al. (2021) advised that performance analysts and coaches should undertake a contextual assessment of the environment. This enables a targeted outcome to change behaviour, facilitate learning, improve efficacy and increase motivation (Groom et al., 2011).

A contextual assessment is an opportunity to consider all factors that may impede the learning experience and facilitation of feedback to athletes. Contextual factors were also raised by Groom et al. (2011). Here, they acknowledged six sub-categories which included social environment, coaching and delivery philosophy, recipient qualities, presentation format, session design and delivery process. Summarising the work of O'Donoghue and Mayes (2013), Groom et al. (2011) and Martin et al. (2021), a brief of factors to consider, prior to communicating performance analysis feedback is listed below.

i Social Environment:

It is important here to consider factors relating to interaction, power and role (Groom et al., 2011) for both the athlete and coach in the delivery of video feedback. It is here, that an assessment must be made on the dynamics within an athlete group as well as the interactions between the coach and athlete, coach and analyst and between analyst and athlete. Martin et al. (2021) suggest performance analysts should prioritise three key roles in the development of relationships, these are: undertake background research, actively build relationships and clearly define roles. A strong coach-analyst/analyst-athlete relationship displays values of openness and honesty (Kojman et al., 2022) as well as characteristics of support and empowerment. As a performance analyst, it is important to remain open-minded, a strong communicator and be self-aware (Robertson, 2020). Of course, we recognise that developing relationships can be challenging, particularly in the early stages. In support, McKenna et al. (2018) suggested a range of ways to support the development of relationships, this might include attending training sessions or travelling to away games and embedding yourself into the environment. These factors can also be used in the development of other significant professional relationships with multidisciplinary support staff.

As well as the role of the analyst, it is also important for athletes to have an understanding of their responsibilities within the feedback process. Here, an evaluation of how individuals interact and relate to each other is needed. Supporting self-awareness, it is also important that athletes, coaches and analysts have an awareness of others and acknowledge how interactions and specifically information communicated in feedback sessions, will make others feel. These interactions are also a factor of the leadership style of the coach. In terms of power, it is important that coaches are aware of the power they may hold on the coach-athlete relationship, and how this may impact interactions.

With sport predominately played on evenings and weekends, Martin et al. (2021) also suggest for analysts to be available to engage with athletes and staff informally. Considering that the majority of preparation for performance debriefs and briefs will be undertaken post-match, contact by athletes and coaches may be received ad hoc. Analyst wellbeing is equally important, so contact hours and method of contact should be discussed in role clarity meetings ensuring performance analysts also have downtime opportunities.

ii Coach philosophy and leadership style:

In the facilitation and communication of feedback the coach's leadership style and philosophy of feedback must be considered (Martin et al., 2021 and Nicholls et al., 2018). The delivery of video-based feedback can be scaffolded depending on what the coach has set out to achieve, for example, whether that be developing winning performances or developing athletes (Groom et al., 2011). Depending on approach, it would impact the construction of clips and the intended delivery style, which would require diligence and time.

Philosophy, known as a guiding principle for behaviour can differ from coach to coach, and equally develop with experience over time. A coach's previous experience of analysis and feedback sessions can impact their philosophy, whether that be in a positive or negative regard. Should a coach have had a positive experience as an athlete, it may reflect in their philosophy and delivery of feedback as a coach. On the contrary, should they have been subject to a negative experience, as acknowledged by Groom et al. (2011), it could impact their appreciation of the service now as a coach. Opposingly, reflective coaches in that situation may wish to create a safe and caring culture which they never received, and an opportunity to facilitate video feedback sessions and valuable learning environments for athletes.

As with philosophy, leadership styles can differ between coaches. Styles, depending on the approach, will dictate the culture within the performance team. Some coaches prefer to be transformational leaders and others opt to be transactional coaches. When considering the communication of feedback, Martin et al. (2021) acknowledged that transactional leaders tended to provide athletes with practical solutions to problems rather than encouraging athletes to work through difficulties, to find their own solutions. The term transactional leader, revealing similar traits to that of an autocratic leader, a term more commonly used in teaching and coaching styles. The alternative transformational approach is seen by O'Donoghue and Mayes (2013) who endorsed the use of online analysis platforms to share footage of performances. This empowers squads and encourages athletes to review and discuss performances online to find their own solutions in the days leading up to the training sessions. Transformational, aligning more so to a democratic teaching and coaching style, whereby a high level of athlete participation is encouraged, giving athletes an involvement in the decision making, goals, practice and performance strategies (Lyle, 2006).

iii Power dynamics:

The phrase 'Power dynamic' refers to the way individuals act or behave, which is influenced by their role. Specifically,

> "social power can be conceived as the resources one person has available so that he or she can influence another person to do what that person would not have done otherwise" (Raven et al., 1998: 307).

In this instance, we will discuss the roles of the coach and athlete in the communication of feedback. Using a model initially developed by French and Raven (1959), redeveloped by Raven (1992) and used Groom et al. (2012), the following stages of power are described:

- **Expert**: The coaches' knowledge that the athlete requires.
- **Referent**: The coach is identifiable as a role model.
- **Information**: The coaches' ability to explain why changed behaviour is preferable
- **Legitimate**: The athlete is expected to comply with the coach's direction.
- **Coercive**: The ability of the coach to discipline an athlete based on non-conformity or behaviour.
- **Reward**: The ability of the coach to reward an athlete based on conformity or behaviour.

O'Donoghue and Mayes (2013), Groom et al. (2011) and Martin et al. (2021) all recognise the importance of power, and the need to observe and identify the dynamics within athlete groups and in relation to coaching teams. Naturally, these characteristics align to the leadership styles and philosophies of coaches communicating feedback. A transformative approach to the coach-athlete relationship, for example, is where positive relationships enabled the provision of performance analysis to flourish (Martin et al., 2021). A secondary example is the two-way communication strand between athletes and coaches, as seen in O'Donoghue and Mayes (2013). These give athletes a sense of ownership and involvement in the decision making of provision, whether that be related to timing of feedback, quantity of information or details of task. Overall, a more conducive and positive learning environment is an equitable power-sharing relationship between coach and athlete (Cassidy et al., 2009).

iv Recipient qualities:

This refers to the coach and the performance analyst having an understanding of the needs and attributes of the athlete or team they are providing feedback to. Essentially, this factor involves developing a best practice framework to meet the needs of individuals, noting that the requirements of individuals may differ to the needs of other team members. This may include the volume of information, the timing and frequency of feedback (Martin et al., 2021), whether they are motivated learners, have a high work ethic or are reflective athletes (Groom et al., 2011). When considering types of feedback sessions, reflect that some athletes may prefer large group sessions and an opportunity to review and reflect on performances publicly, consistently engaging in dialogue with peers and coaches. On the other hand, the preference of other athletes would be to review performances in a one-to-one setting with an opportunity to ask questions or post comments to online clips in a safe and private platform. In large group sessions, these individuals may remain reserved and whilst they are quietly engaged, they may refrain from speaking publicly due to factors such as confidence, nervousness or due to wider factors such as athlete power dynamics.

Another factor which needs consideration when communicating feedback is non-visible disabilities. These are often oversighted unless the performance analyst or coach has a strong understanding of individual athlete needs. Examples of non-visible disabilities include hearing loss and dyslexia and whilst colour blindness is not recognised as a disability, it can impact individuals interpreting colours on charts, dashboards and videos. This is by no means an exhaustive list of non-visible disabilities, but consider the scenario below and how it may impact the three athletes with non-visible disabilities.

> *The coach and performance analyst have developed a group feedback session for twenty athletes following Saturday's performance. In preparation for the session, the coach and performance analyst have created a playlist of video clips reflecting their strengths with further clips highlighting areas that need development. The role of the athlete in this session is to review the playlist (red team versus green team), discuss with the athlete sitting next to you and then provide two comments each on the white board at the back of the room. Actions will be taken into the training session straight after analysis.*

Naively and unaware of the recipient's needs, the scenario above may seem a productive way to deliver feedback prior to training. Yet, based on the needs of the three individuals with non-visible disabilities, some approaches should be considered.

- **Hearing loss**: Consider the delivery setting of an analysis session for an individual with hearing loss. Despite having the ability to lipread conversations, a large group session situated in a computer room could be troublesome. First, with multiple ongoing conversations and second with individuals working behind computer monitors, the opportunity to lipread becomes challenging. A smaller group setting with less simultaneous conversations might be a more comfortable environment.

- **Colour Blindness:** Review the use of complementary analysis tools that can be incorporated to enhance the delivery of feedback and support an individual with colour blindness. In this situation whereby colours cannot be clearly recognised, consider the use of annotations or voiceovers on video sequences. By including shapes or labels on video clips, it can support an individual identifying the area for discussion.
- **Dyslexia:** Reflect on the feedback method on completion of the analysis task. Whilst this is completed to check and challenge athlete understanding, the task of writing on a white board in front of others may cause some individual's discomfort. This is an environment where they feel they will make mistakes or can be made to feel foolish in front of peers and coaches based on their writing, spelling or communication of a word. As an alternative, could the task be conducted in pairs and a peer lead on the administrative task, or in place of written notes could a verbal summary be provided in the classroom or later sent using audio notes.

Delivery Approach

O'Donoghue and Mayes (2013) and Groom et al. (2011) both acknowledged a cyclical approach to the delivery of video-based feedback. This incorporates a train, game and review process whereby goals are consistently reviewed. O'Donoghue and Mayes (2013), who specifically focused on the observe, reflect, plan and act process, identified a clear connection between each phase which in turn highlights a continuous learning cycle. This is demonstrated in the communication about video clips phase, which leads into the pre-training discussion and then squad training. This suggests a **review** to **practice** approach, where learnings from video reviews discussed either in online analysis platforms or in classroom will then be actioned in a live training environment. Regardless of the feedback stage (training, competition, post-performance), consider the contextual factors discussed above and how these may support the infrastructure of delivering feedback. This may include empowering athletes by having an equitable power-share and engaging individuals or the leadership group in the decisions related to the delivery of feedback (Martin et al., 2021). It is important to note that these individuals are the stakeholders in this process and so the type, timing and quantity of information should be suitable to their requirements and as the recipients of the information, these individuals are best placed to advise on their requests. A bespoke feedback design promoting discussion, athlete reflection, empowerment and ownership of analysis can then be implemented (Martin et al., 2021).

Having said this, care must be taken by the performance analyst and coach in this situation, first by managing the expectations of athletes that all requests may not be feasible and second by ensuring the power-share remains balanced. It is in environments such as this, that athlete demands may become overbearing and a shift in power towards athletes and away from coaches may be seen.

a Training

Of course, it is natural to assume that certain environments will provide a greater opportunity to deliver and communicate feedback with athletes and coaches. Environments, such as training, are deemed more flexible whereby performance analysts, coaches and athletes can interact more freely. It is in these environments that performance analysts have an opportunity to deliver a live review of tasks undertaken which supports training. There are a number of ways in which this can be conducted, from setting up a live sharing platform, to simply connecting a feed from the performance analyst station to a TV at the side of the training facility. In either approach and depending on the environment, it provides an opportunity for athletes and coaches to engage in a conversation and confirm performance structures prior to reattempting the required skill.

Should facilitating live reviews at training environments not be feasible, due to the sport, facility or equipment available, filming the session to review later is just as beneficial. This can also be used to inform future training sessions and discussions. Whilst the footage cannot be reviewed immediately or between drills, it is in situations like these, that coach and athlete interactions can be captured. Verbal and non-verbal directions given by the coach can be observed by the athlete away from training and in a phase of reflection and checking of role clarity.

b Competition

Communication of feedback during a performance can be impacted by the sport itself and also the rules. With sports that have natural breaks in performance, such as between games, rounds, sets, quarters and half time periods, the delivery of feedback can be more streamlined. This is an opportunity for coaches to provide feedback with an intent to immediately impact the ongoing performance. With sports that are continuous or cyclical, the delivery of feedback can be more troublesome. For example, in events which are categorised as races (swimming, cycling or running), feedback is more commonly received at the conclusion of the event. Yet, it's not so straightforward, even feedback opportunities for these events can fluctuate, for example, there may be opportunity to quickly interact with an athlete in a long-distance race, albeit the event will continue. Naturally, with short distance races and the time taken to complete these events, this would not be feasible.

In terms of type and quantity of feedback, this will depend on the athlete's needs, the coach's leadership style and the time given between performance periods. Within the rules of squash, athletes are provided with a 90-second interval between games, whilst at international level netball players receive a 4-minute break between quarters and a 12-minute interval at half time. Performance periods range for each sport; some sports also have opportunities to pause play using water breaks, this giving coaches a chance to provide additional information from pitch or court side.

The method of communicating feedback during play at an elite level, will also vary from sport to sport. Rugby union for example Presents or displays a strong connection between performance analyst and coach who are frequently seen working collaboratively in a coaching box in the stands of the stadium. This is an opportunity for coaches to review footage and discuss tactical strategies based on the data prior to communicating with athletes in half time breaks. Alternatively, in elite level soccer, a coach or manager can be found in the pitch side technical area. Until early 2018, soccer coaches were expected to direct, instruct and make tactical changes without analysis support. In July 2018, the International Football Association Board (www.theifab.com) announced an amendment to the laws of the game, permitting small hand-held electronic or communication devices for use in coaching and tactics in the technical area. This rule change also permits an analyst to relocate to the technical area to present data or video clips to coaches from feeds around the stadium.

As raised previously, time constraints play a large factor in the communication of feedback during organised intervals (quarter or half time breaks). Largely, the coach and management team will have a pre-planned strategy of what this period will look like. This could involve a summary to the entire team led by the head coach, before athletes break into small groups based on their position to discuss specific elements with a technical attack or defence coach. Depending on the coach's wishes, this may involve the delivery of objective data to affirm the feedback points raised (for example, the total number of turnovers gained and scored in netball). In other sports, whereby a coach is seen to be working closely with an analyst during performance, one or two clips could be identified in readiness to be shared with individuals, positional units or, if relevant, with the entire team during the half time break in the team's changing room.

c Post-Competition

On the completion of data collection and the generation of results, feedback can be shared with athletes and coaches in preparation for debrief (review) sessions. A tool used by performance teams to facilitate self-correction, develop team cohesion and improve future performances (Kojman et al., 2022). Sessions can be developed upon four key components: (1) self-reflection of the performances in terms of strengths and areas to develop, (2) visionary aids supporting coach and athlete discussion, (3) identification and confirmation of strategy changes and (4) the setting of goals (Hogg, 2002). In covering these components, a meeting time and place, duration of session and balance of information all need to be considered, aligning to the competition environment.

Depending on situation and sport, a performance analyst may have the fortunate opportunity of delivering a debrief of Saturday's fixture on a Monday whilst facilitating a preview of the next fixture on a Thursday. Whilst the balance of information and timing of these sessions is still vitally important, sessions can be segregated allowing athletes time to reflect on what has happened, prior to engaging in an opposition review on what to expect next. Other sports or competition environments may not be so forgiving, with multiple matches scheduled in a short competition window. Depending on the sport, this could involve two performances in one day or back-to-back fixtures on consecutive days. In this instance, the timing and balance of information in a feedback session would need attention. In this example, an evening fixture may need debriefing immediately post-performance, followed immediately by a preview meeting for a fixture the following lunchtime. The briefing meeting is usually organised to take place on the same evening as performance one rather than on the morning of performance two. This ensures that there is enough time given to athletes to digest the information prior to performing but also safeguarding athlete preparation time and performance routines on the morning of a fixture. Should back-to-back sessions take place, it would be advised to take a short break between debrief and briefing meetings. This could be a short drink break or a quick preorganised team activity; ultimately, the aim is to give athletes an opportunity to switch off and then refocus their attention for the next session.

Regardless of the post-match feedback format, it is important that athletes are aware of their role and have an understanding of the purpose and intent of sessions. Ultimately, the delivery of feedback is to support athlete development in a bid to improve future performances. Within the feedback process, it is important that athletes adopt an open mindset and showcase the qualities of honesty and integrity (Groom et al., 2011). Their engagement in this process as motivated learners will support their ability to update knowledge and behaviours whilst understanding their own performance standards in a safe space (Kojman, 2022). Similarly, the coach and performance analyst must also understand their roles within the delivery process, being mindful that the misuse of video can negatively impact athlete engagement and development.

Below are examples (i–iv) of post-performance feedback methods, which can be employed depending on environments, skill level, gender and age of recipients and stakeholders in feedback sessions.

i Hot debrief

Hot debrief is a term used to review performances in an emotionally charged atmosphere (Kojman, 2022). This is usually undertaken at the performance venue, immediately after performing. With emotions high regardless of the result, it is important that the coach provides objective data, detaching from subjective emotions that may cloud viewpoints. In this instance, the coach would require a set of key performance indicator results from the performance analyst immediately post-performance. For this environment, it is likely that indicators have been pre-arranged and confirmed by coaches and athlete leadership group. With this, the performance analyst will either have an output window prepared which can generate results immediately on the completion of performance or if data has been shared to coaches using an electronic device (tablet or laptop) during the performance, results will already be available. Despite the approach, a schedule would have been confirmed between performance analyst and coach, for when and how the output window will be received in readiness for the hot debrief. This may be a simple text message or email direct to a mobile phone, or it may have been arranged that the performance analyst facilitates the session itself. These are all discussion points that should have been raised at the clarity and expectations meeting at the commencement of the season. Whilst video plays a key part in debriefing sessions, it is unlikely due to time, recovery schedules and possibly travel that video will feature in these immediate hot-brief sessions.

ii 1-1 or Unit debriefs

Depending on sport or environment, some coaches may offer the opportunity to communicate feedback in a 1:1 setting, or should it be more convenient, feedback may be delivered to athletes in smaller groups or as positional units. The benefit of these sessions is that athletes have an opportunity to discuss personal roles and responsibilities without the judgements of the wider team. To support these sessions, a coach may ask an athlete or unit to select a series of clips on a related topic and bring to the meeting. This not only provides an opportunity for coaches to check an athlete's understanding of the topic area, but it also provides an athlete with an opportunity to gain clarity on performance roles. Whilst this may be a time-consuming task for coaches, who in rugby union can have up to 15 starting players, it can provide an opportunity for athletes who rarely contribute to group discussions an opportunity to be heard. Smaller group meetings such as these, are examples of coaches scaffolding learning opportunities. Often using video-feedback and questioning, these types of sessions can aid athlete learning and development of tactical knowledge (Middlemas et al., 2018; McRobert & Williams, 2019).

iii Team debriefs

Team debriefs are an opportunity to review performances as whole. This is a useful time saving task, whereby information presented to an individual or unit might be beneficial to another. In that case, having all parties present ensures that a consistent message is received by all. In terms of delivering these sessions, they do become more constructed and streamlined over time. This is a result of gaining experience and becoming more confident in the role. As an analyst, whether your responsibility is to lead the video feedback session or to facilitate the session along with a coach, it is an opportunity to share knowledge and give clarity to performance situations.

Whilst the session is labelled as a team debrief, the way in which these are structured will depend on the teaching preferences of the coach and the aims of the session. This will influence the design of the session, which can vary from a solo coach delivery, a review in units or a complete player-led session (Middlemas et al., 2018). Of course, the success of sessions impinges on athlete engagement; their willingness to honestly and critically reflect on performance. Presentation designs (video clips, annotations, slide designs, in session tasks and take-home tasks) all have a part to play in athlete engagement and 'landing the feedback' message. A well prepared and slick production, combining performance indicators and the presentation of videos which are played in full screen and delivered within the time constraints of the scheduled session, will certainly be favoured, over messy and unorganised presentations.

Depending on the autocratic or democratic coaching style displayed by a coach and the learning preferences of the participants (behaviourism, constructivism and cognitivism), the session can be delivered very differently. Mosston and Ashworth (2008) introduced the spectrum of teaching styles, which in this case has been applied to performance analysis debrief sessions. The spectrum is designed across a continuum, with opposing ideologies at either end focusing on either, a) coach led pedagogies or b) player-led pedagogies. Coach led pedagogies is separated by two extremes. Firstly, **command** (style A) which is solely a coach led delivery, and secondly, **inclusion (**style E), which suggests tasks are created by the coach for athletes to decide on what meets their ability. A further three styles (B to D) are situated between these. Contrastingly, at the other end of the spectrum, focus is transferred to player-led pedagogies. This is firstly categorised by **guided discovery** (style F) which as suggested by its letter is situated along from inclusion. In this instance, a coach provides a task for athletes to source a solution that was not previously known. The continuum then moves towards, **self-teaching** (style K), which is the development of knowledge without guided or formal instruction. Naturally, the teaching preferences of coaches and the learning preferences of athletes will dictate which approach is delivered and the types of tasks included.

Video has now become extremely accessible (Kojman, 2022) and is a powerful tool in the facilitation of feedback. As noted previously, it presents visual aids to assist coach and athlete discussions to support learning, and is commonly used in team debrief meetings regardless of coaching style preferences. Yet, the selection of video sequences is now becoming more critical. With research indicating a preference that debrief session decrease from 40 minutes (Groom and Cushion, 2005) to 20 minutes or less (Nicholls et al., 2018), a greater allocation of time is needed in the planning and construction of a comprehensive presentation. With time a factor, coaches may wish to facilitate a culture whereby athletes take responsibility and conduct self-analysis away from training environments

(O'Donoghue and Mayes, 2013), with athletes bringing personal or unit playlists to these larger settings to facilitate discussions with teammates and coaches.

In a wider setting, time can also be precious for performance analysts in the management of workloads to meet pressing presentation deadlines. Video content and objective data will be required for team debrief sessions but the next steps can then depend on the personal preferences of the analyst and equally the amount of time readily available. Using the scenario above of having two back-to-back performances on consecutive days, the construction of video resources will need to be well-planned and organised, allowing presentations to be delivered promptly post-performance. In this instance preparation is key, and this can be helped with the development of supporting resources in advance of competition. This can include the design and construction of slide decks, which include the team branding and colours, opposition name and logo, date and place of fixture and slide titles in readiness for video sequences. Then depending on preference, performance analysts may wish to develop their presentation within the performance analysis package itself. As an example, both Hudl SportsCode (HUDL, Lincoln, NE) and Nacsport (Nacsport, Gran Canaria, Spain) provide the capability of developing presentations and importing of slide decks to customise workflows. Alternatively, some performance analysts may wish to select and export their video clips from the performance analysis package and import sequences into a presentation platform such as PowerPoint or Keynote. The strength of option A is that the presentation is housed in one platform, meaning the additional step to export video clips is not required. Depending on time constraints, this might be a convenient solution. The benefit of option B is that the presentation can be shared immediately with coaches and athletes (once videos have been exported from the analysis platform), and it can be played without the requirement of specialised software. Of course, a presentation developed in an analysis platform can be shared, yet the recipient will either need to have the specialist software on their own machine for it to play or the presentation will need to be exported as a standalone video.

iv Online sharing platforms

Moving towards a player-led pedagogy, the use of online platforms has become increasingly more popular with performance teams and sports. The capability for performance footage to be uploaded and shared to a password protected site, usually managed by the performance analyst has advanced the communication of feedback. Whilst O'Donoghue and Mayes (2013) acknowledged their existence, they have developed instrumentally with the competition of platforms greater than ever. These video sharing platforms enhance the coaching process allowing a greater volume of feedback to be provided to individuals (O'Donoghue and Mayes (2013)), who have the capability to review and comment on clips at a time and place convenient to them. Platforms such as HUDL Online (HUDL, Lincoln, NE), Coach Logic (Coach Logic, Edinburgh, UK) and In-Play Sports (In-Play Sports, Doncaster, UK) are just a few examples of the online market. These platforms provide teams with an online video storage capacity depending on the level of subscription purchased. Admin users, such as the performance analyst, then have the capability of managing the upload and archiving of footage and playlists to ensure adequate capacity is always available. Admin users are also provided the ability to manage user access, which involves the enrolment of new athletes or coaches using an email address.

A benefit of online sharing platforms is not only the access to performance footage but also access to the coded timeline created by the performance analyst. A timeline which lasts the duration of the match, marked up with indicators of when events occurred (see Chapter 5). The timeline coincides with key performance indicators generated and provides an opportunity to review set events without the need to review the entire match. Post-performance and on conclusion of data collection, the performance analyst can upload footage with an XML document directly to the secure online platform. Here, access can be provided for certain users (e.g., defenders, coaches), depending on the relevance of the footage. HUDL online also has the capability for users to create their own or add to an existing playlist which can be shared with all or just selected users. Within presentation playlists, users (athletes and coaches) have the opportunity to communicate through comments and draw on clips using annotations. This is an opportunity for athletes to gain clarity on performance actions, receive feedback from teammates and coaches on points raised and have a visual record of events easily accessible from a mobile phone app or web browser for future confirmation. As with team debriefs, coaches may also opt to prepare and construct a brief or debrief playlist online rather than within the performance analysis specialised software. The playlist is then accessible for athletes to review on multiple machines in unit or team debriefs. With teams likely to have a minimum number for specialised software licences, the use of online sharing platforms provides an opportunity for complete timelines to be shared and be accessible to subscribed users via any internet browser.

Conclusions

The role and responsibilities of a performance analyst in the communication of feedback is not clear cut, with factors such as learning and teaching preferences needing consideration. With styles interchangeable, it is important to develop an appreciation and understanding of all. As an example, *what might work now, may not work under new management.* So, in summary, a performance analyst toolbox has been created below:

Relationship building

Regardless of personnel or styles, the development of relationships with stakeholders is key to success. It is important to not solely focus of the development of hard-skills, but spend quality time developing a soft-skill toolkit. This may include qualities such as: interpersonal skills, self-awareness, communication skills, negotiation skills, creativity in the delivery and design of presentations and time management.

Feedback strategy

Collaborate with coaches and athletes to design and develop a feedback strategy which captures the needs of the stakeholders (Martin et al., 2021). Stakeholder buy-in is key, this ensuring the strategy is fit for purpose, whilst ensuring all parties are involved in the decision making. Although be conscious that an equitable power balance is managed.

Preparation

Preparation and adaptability characteristics are key to a thriving performance analyst, particularly in the communication of feedback. The design and development of supporting materials ahead of fixtures can ease the pressure in competition environments. These can then be used to supplement objective data and video sequences collected, in creating athlete learning resources.

Delivery

To create a conducive and enjoyable feedback environment, it is important to design athlete engaging resources which are presented in a timely manner. These resources must be appropriate for the environment (training, brief or debrief) with the performance analyst effectively managing access to shared online resources (performance footage and playlists). Evaluating delivery methods is also advised (Martin et al., 2021). Firstly, this can be achieved by capturing the experiences of the recipients of the feedback environment. Plus, a self-reflection of the experience can be conducted by noting thoughts and feelings of the events and generating an action plan for future practices (Gibbs, 1988).

9 Performance profiles

Introduction

This chapter discusses profiling in sports performance analysis, covering developments in profiles over time, different types of profiles and examples of their use. This chapter covers profiles of individual performances as well as profiles of typical performance that use data from multiple matches. The profiles are presented as both radar charts and line graphs allowing a critical comparison of these representations. The profiles also compare the use of absolute performance indicator values and relative performance which relates performance to the relevant population of performances.

The meaning of the word "profiling"

The term performance profiling was first introduced in sports performance analysis by Hughes et al. (2001) to describe a method to determine the number of performances required for a performance variable to stabilise within a tolerable limit of its true mean. This could be done for a single performer of interest or data from multiple performers could be used to produce profile deriving a given type of performance. A single performer could be a team or an individual player for whom we have a data on a large set of performances. This set of performances may not be every performance ever completed by the performer. Therefore, we refer to this set of performances as a sample. The technique of Hughes et al. (2001) was applied to performance variables in isolation. The mean of the variable was determined as an estimate of the true mean for the given performer. The technique then analysed subsamples of increasing size by adding each value in turn. The percentage difference between the subsample mean and the sample mean (as an estimate of the true mean) was calculated as the subsample grew. Eventually, when all of the values were added, there would be no difference between these two means. Hughes et al. (2001) observed the minimum number of values needed for the percentage difference to fall within some tolerable limit and remain within these limits as the remaining values are added. These limits could be 5% or 10% for example. Some performance variables are more stable than others

DOI: 10.4324/9781003375463-9

and require fewer values for the subsample mean to fall within the tolerable percentage difference to the sample mean than other variables. For example, the number of passes in a team game would typically be a more stable variable than the number of shots. The same process could be applied to data from multiple performers where a research study was being done and the researchers wanted to provide a rationale for the sample size they were using in terms of the stability of the data.

Determining the number of performances needed for variables to stabilise within tolerable limits of the estimated true mean has merit in practical performance analysis and in academic research (Parson et al., 2001; Vivian et al., 2001). However, Hughes et al. (2001) used the terms "profile" and "profiling" differently to the way these terms have been used in other disciplines of sports science as well as other fields outside sport. The Cambridge Dictionary (2022) provides the following meanings for the word profile when it is used as a verb:

- "to write or publish a short description of someone's life, work, character, etc."
- "to predict the likely behaviour or description of someone such as a customer or criminal, based on what information you have about them"
- "to give a short description of someone or something with important and useful details about them"

It is the second and third meanings, listed here, that represent the way "profiling" and "profiles" are used in academic and professional settings. Later, in this chapter, we will consider the first of these meanings though. It is fair to say that profiles in sports performance analysis describe performance rather but not to the extent that future performances could be accurately predicted. The third meaning from the Cambridge Dictionary characterises very well how profiles have been used in sports science. Let us consider the fitness profiles and the profiles that are used in sports psychology. Fitness profiles (Sedano et al., 2009) provide a "short description" that is an abstract representation of fitness, perhaps summarising it a 6–12 key fitness variables. These fitness variables are the "important and useful details" representing different aspects of fitness such as strength, power, endurance, speed, flexibility and co-ordination. Some published research studies use the term "physiological profiles" where maximal oxygen consumption is included but still include fitness test results and anthropometric variables (McIntyre and Hall, 2005). Profiles in sports psychology are also collections of variables that form an abstract representation of broad complex concepts of interest. For example, the profile of mood states (POMS) summarises mood with abstract numerical variables representing the dimensions of anger, confusion, depression, fatigue, tension and vigour (McNair et al., 1971). The Competitive State Anxiety Inventory-2 (CSAI-2) is an abstract representation of the complexity of anxiety in sport that includes the intensity and direction of worry, somatic anxiety and concentration disruption (Martens et al., 1990; Mellalieu et al., 2004). The term "performance profile" has been used extensively in sports psychology (Butler and Hardy, 1992; Butler, 1996; Gucciardi and Gordon, 2009).

The reason for providing "short descriptions" that cover the "important and useful details" is to improve our understanding of the person or group being profiled. Having a clear understanding of performance is an aim of performance analysis in general. Clear understanding of areas of performance requiring attention informs decisions about preparation for forthcoming competition. Therefore, the way in which the important details within a profile should be presented needs to consider best way to convey the information to the intended audience. Graphical representation is a way of presenting profiles that have been used in management profiles (Quinn et al., 1996). Quinn et al. (1996) used a radar chart to display eight different management roles on a backdrop showing ideal optimal scores for these. This representation allows the viewer to immediately see areas where engagement with roles is too low or high to be positive as well as areas where there is optimal engagement. Related roles were grouped within neighbouring sectors of the radar chart which meant that the viewer not only interprets engagement in the roles in isolation but also sees the broader pattern of management style. It was Quinn et al.'s (1996) profiling technique used in management that had the largest influence on O'Donoghue's (2005) profiling technique used in sports performance analysis. The remainder of this chapter will discuss profiles of sports performance and the collections of variables they include.

Measurement issues in profiling

Validity

There are four measurement issues of concern to profiles in sports performance analysis; validity, objectivity, reliability and stability. A profile can be fundamentally compromised if the variables within the profile lack relevance or have been measured inaccurately. It must be noted, however, that this is not an issue with any profiling technique. The profiling techniques are intended to be used with good quality data, but there is no doubt that it is possible for somebody to create a profile containing invalid and unreliable variables. There is no difference here to using a statistical technique with poor quality data. The issue is not with the t test, analysis of variance test, correlation or nonparametric test as techniques. The issue is that these statistical techniques have been applied to data that are open to criticism. So hopefully the reader understands that it is not the role of a profiling technique to establish the validity, objectivity and reliability of the variables used within the profile. It is expected, however, that the techniques will be used to create profiles containing high quality variables and that the data represented have been gathered in a diligent manner.

We will start with validity. The variables within a performance profile should represent important and relevant aspects of sports performance that are useful to coaches and players. A variable has logical validity, sometime referred to as face validity, where it obviously represents the aspect of performance of interest. For example, the times and distances achieved by heptathletes and decathletes for the running, jumping and throwing disciplines within these multi-event sports. Criterion validity is where a performance indicator is associated with overall performance outcome. For example, a performance indicator may have a strong correlation with the margin of victory in a rugby union match. Logical validity and criterion validity are relevant to the individual variables included within a performance profile. The type of validity that is of most relevance to profiles is content validity. Content validity for performance profiles can be seen the same way that it is seen for a questionnaire. Consider a questionnaire about spectator experience at sports events. The questionnaire has content validity if the questions cover all of the subtopics that are relevant to spectator experience. For example, it should include variables for quality of entertainment, cost of attendance, viewing position, atmosphere, merchandise, refreshments, travel to the venue, parking and timing of sports events. Similarly, a performance profile should include variables representing all of the important aspects of performance. For example, in an invasive field game, we would represent shooting, passing, possession, territory, defending, set pieces, off-the-ball movement, discipline and aerial play depending on the sport. When we say that a performance profile needs to represent all of the relevant aspects of performance in the sport to have content validity, we need to consider that some sports are so complex that we may have different profiles for different aspects. For example, the performance indicators that are relevant to players and units within teams may need to be position-specific (James et al., 2005). There may be different coaches within a squad for different areas of performance, for example, goalkeeping coaches in soccer. Performance profiles should be appropriate for the coaches and athletes who will be using the information. This is important to ensuring that profiles are manageable for their users.

Consider the match statistics that are provided by IBM Slam Tracker on the US Open website (US Open, 2021a). Specifically, we will consider the final of the 2021 women's singles at the US Open between Emma Raducanu and Leylah Fernandez. The basic statistics for this match form a profile, all-be-it a profile for a single match. Indeed, it could be considered as two separate profiles, one for the performance of each player. These basic statistics include variables for point outcomes when serving and receiving, aces, double faults, net points, break points, winners, unforced errors and distance covered. Some of these statistics are raw frequencies and others show percentages of points that are successful. When one clicks on "full stats", it is possible to see these same variables for the individual sets within the match. There are other tabs allowing serve statistics, return statistics, rally statistics and service direction statistics to be displayed. All of this information could be considered to be excessive for a profile, but the website has the benefit of being interactive so that the user can navigate to the subset of statistics of most interest to them.

A performance indicator is a variable that is valid, with an objective measurement process, a known measurement scale and a valid means of interpretation (Bevan, 1995). In order to be able to interpret the performance indicator, we need to know what values are considered high, average or low for the performance indicator and whether good performance is represented by high, low or medium values. Performance profiles add an extra element to the interpretation of performance indicators where performance indicators are considered together. When viewing the profile, the coach, player or analyst can consider all variables together when interpreting serving performance. The English Institute of Sport takes this further with the "What It Takes To Win" (WITTW) approach (EIS, 2021) where different elements of performance contributing to outcome are identified. These elements of performance are associated with the fitness, technical, tactical and other abilities required to achieve the levels of performance necessary in the elements to deliver a winning outcome.

Objectivity

As already mentioned in Chapter 2, some variables in sports performance are more "matter of fact" than others. The objectivity of a performance indicator depends on the objectivity with which individual match events can be classified. This requires an objective measurement procedure so that those collecting performance data are doing so correctly and those using the information know what the values mean. Where variables are not so matter-of-fact and open to interpretation, we can demonstrate a level of objectivity through inter-operator agreement studies. Where a measurement process can be applied consistently by different operators we achieve a good level of inter-operator agreement.

While objectivity is primarily an issue for the individual variables included within a performance profile, there are some occasions where we need to be objective about the profile itself. For example, where a profile leads to an overall score for the performance, we need to understand how variables within the profile combined to provide us with this score. For example, in multi-event sports like the heptathlon, decathlon and modern pentathlon, there are formal equations for converting times and distances into points that are then added to determine the overall points score for the performance (Dinnie and O'Donoghue, 2020).

One of the main differences between variables in sports performance analysis and other disciplines of sports science is that the other disciplines have standard variables. For example, multiple studies will have used standard tests such as the Wingate test (Vandewalle et al., 1987) or instruments such as

POMS (McNair et al., 1971). Some tests and instruments may have different variants or protocols, but most often users can reference a published source for the specific version. Sports performance analysis is very different with studies continually introducing new variables to represent aspects of sports of interest to the researchers. Some of these variables are very specific not only to a particular aspect of the sport but also to a particular playing style or philosophy. The defensive and offensive positive and negative counts and defensive balance variables used by the Norwegian Football Association (Olsen and Larsen, 1997) are examples of this. This requires specific attention to reliability to be demonstrated for the new variables. There are some standards emerging, such as Opta's match variables in soccer (StatsPerform, 2022), the widely used CricInfo system in cricket (espn, 2022) and DataVolley in volleyball (DataVolley, 2022). The understanding of performance profiles could be enhanced if they used standard variables. Williams has argued the need for consensus about the sets of performance indicators to be used to represent performance in different sports and for the definitions of these performance indicators (Williams, 2012).

Reliability

Reliability is related to objectivity and validity. A variable cannot be valid if it is measured so inconsistently that we don't know what the values mean. While demonstrating good objectivity through good inter-operator agreement is possible in the absence of rigorous operational definitions, there remains a threat to reliability without well understood definitions of variables or at least guidance as to the events represented by the variables. Limited reliability can be a threat to profiles where some data are clearly problematic while other data may have been reliably gathered. Let us consider the serve direction statistics in the 2021 US Open tennis second round women's singles match between Emma Raducanu and Shuai Zhang (US Open, 2021b). According to these statistics, both players served to the outside third of both the deuce and advantage service box on both first and second serve in every service point. This is very unlikely, especially for the second serve which players would tend to play safer than the first serve. Even with the first serve, there is a danger that an opponent will anticipate serve direction if all serves are placed in the same third of the service box. These values could have resulted from a misunderstanding of how to enter the data with third of the service box being confused with which service box was being served to. Alternatively, an operator may have entered all of the service directions the same way thinking no-one would ever look at these statistics because neither player would make the final; oops! Perhaps the match was a genuine outlier where both players served as stated in the match statistics? A quick look at a short highlights video of the match (US Open, 2021c) will discount this theory. In a situation like this where there is a clear reliability issue with data, the match should not be included in the set of matches used to create a profile for a given player or team. Indeed, we would need to have sufficient evidence from a subset of remaining matches that the serve direction variables are reliable if these variables are to be included in a profile.

Stability

Stability is a measurement issue that specifically relates to sports performance variables. The distinction between stability and reliability is that stability is to do with genuine variability in a player's or team's performances. The data for each performance may have been gathered 100% reliably but there may be variability between performances, or even within performances, due to situational variables or random variability. The main situational variable influencing sports performance is the quality of opposition (McGarry and Franks, 1994) with venue (Tenga et al., 2010) and scoreline (Lago, 2009) being found to influence performances in other studies. This variability in sports performance is a characteristic of sports performance that O'Donoghue (2005) wished to represent within his profiling technique. Some performers may be more consistent than others. Some performers may be consistent in some aspects of their performance but inconsistent in other aspects. Rather than trying to determine a number of matches needed to stabilise a performance indicator's mean within tolerable limits of the estimated true mean, O'Donoghue (2005) decided not to stabilise inherently inconsistent performance. The existence of variability in sports performance has been studied further in soccer (Gregson et al., 2010), basketball throws (Coves et al., 2020), technical and physical performance in basketball (Mateus et al., 2015), tactical effectiveness in soccer (Dos Reis and Almeida, 2020) and game actions in volleyball (Ramos et al., 2017).

A profile of typical performance

Pre-processing performance variables

Figure 9.1 summarises tennis performances for a fictitious player in a tournament where matches are the best of three sets. The profile is based on all matches the player completed at the given tournament. This profile has been created using O'Donoghue's (2005) approach which relates performance indicators to the norms for the particular level of the sport. For example, consider the points won on serve when the player's first serve was in (%Won 1st) during matches within the tournament. These are firstly dimensionalised into the percentage of points won when the first serve was in. The reason for this is that some tennis matches are longer than others and so a raw frequency of points won on first serve may give a misleading representation of the serving performance. For example, the player could win 20 points on first serve in the first match and 30 points on first serve in the second match. However, the player may have played 25 points where the first serve was in during the

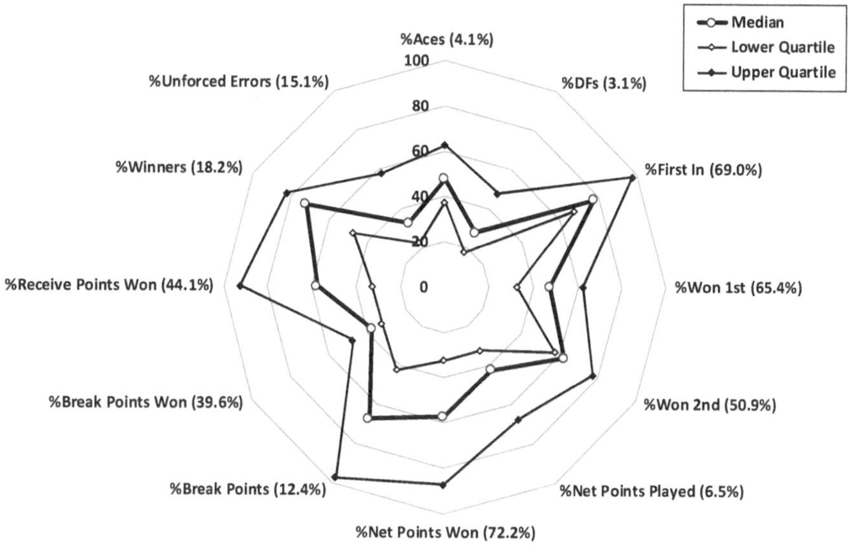

Figure 9.1 A profile of fictitious player's performances in a tennis tournament.

first match and 60 such points in the second match. Thus, the percentage of points that were won when the first serve was in would be 80% and 50%, respectively. Similar pre-processing should be applied to the other variables to adjust for the different number of serving, receiving and net points played in each match.

Reflecting on 2005

O'Donoghue (2005) wanted to represent any consistent and inconsistent areas of performance within profiles. In the original paper, the mean performance was used to represent typical performance and the interquartile range was used to represent the spread of performances about this average. The use of the mean (often used when parametric procedures are applied) and the interquartile range (often used when nonparametric procedures are applied) raised a few eyebrows. So why was this done? This decision was made during the analysis of 28 performances by Venus Williams where it was originally intended to use the mean and the standard deviation. There was one variable where the mean plus one standard deviation exceeded 100% which is obviously impossible for a percentage variable. This suggests that the variable was skewed or asymmetrically distributed with more spread below the mean than above the mean. A test of normality actually found the variable to be sufficiently normal for parametric procedures to be applied. Therefore, there was a great desire to use the mean because it was derived from all 28 values. The median could take any value as long as the value was between the 14th and the 15th when the values were arranged in ascending order. Displaying the spread of performances as ranging from the mean minus one standard deviation to the mean plus one standard deviation was a non-starter due to upper limit of this range exceeding 100%. So, the interquartile range was used to ensure the lower and upper quartiles were within the range of values recorded for the player. The combination of mean and interquartile range can be justified by the fact that the profile did not claim the distribution of values was normally distributed or otherwise and no inferential tests making assumptions about the distribution of values were applied. However, in hindsight, it may have been better to use the median and the interquartile range in the Venus Williams example in O'Donoghue's (2005) paper. Alternatively, the mean could have been used with a spread of performances equivalent to 0.67 standard deviations. This spread would represent the middle 50% of performances if the data were normally distributed. However, even where the data satisfy tests of normality, this does not mean the data are perfectly normal. Also, the interquartile range is an easier concept to explain to practitioners than the standard deviation let alone why the standard deviation is being multiplied by 0.67.

Using quantiles

So back to Figure 9.1 and the profile for our fictitious tennis player. The player's median value for the percentage points won when the first serve was in (%Won 1st) is 65.4%. The middle 50% of the players' performances for this variable has values ranging from the lower quartile of 61.0% to the upper quartile of 69.%. This seems to be reasonably symmetrical about the median. However, it is not obvious whether this interquartile range represents consistent or inconsistent performance for this variable. Therefore, this profiling technique (O'Donoghue, 2005) did not plot the values for the performance variables, but instead plotted the percentage of players in the relevant population that the median, lower and upper quartiles exceeded. This is an approach that has been used with body mass index where percentiles have been published for different ages and genders by the National Centre for Chronic Disease Prevention and Health Promotion (NCCDPHP, 2000). The percentiles drawn on the chart were for 5%, 10%, 25%, 50%, 75%, 85%, 90% and 95%. This allows someone to look at a chart for their gender, find their age on the horizontal axis, body mass index on the vertical axis and see what percentile banding they are in for their age and gender.

The full set of matches in the given tournament can be used to determine vigintile norms for this level, age group, and gender of tennis performers. Vigintile norms split a set of values into 20 groups each representing roughly 5% of the population of values. There are 19 of these values from the 5% to the 95% percentiles. These 19 values can split data into 20 groups just as three quartiles (the 25%, 50% and 75% percentiles) can split data into four groups. The player's median value for the percentage of points won when the first serve was in (65.4%) sits in the 10th of the 20 5% bandings, between the 45% and 50% percentiles. Thus, the player's median performance is in the 5% of performances such that 45% of performances see a lower percentage of points won on first serve and 50% of performances see a higher percentage of points won on first serve. The player's lower quartile for this variable (61.0%) sits in the 7th of the 20 5% bandings (between the 30% and 35% percentiles) indicating that the top three quarters of the player's performances for percentage of points won when the first serve is in are located in the top 70% of performances one sees at this level of tennis. The player's upper quartile for this variable (69.8%) is in the 13th of the 20 5% bandings indicating that the player's best 25% of performances for this variable are located in the best 35% of performances for the relevant population of performances.

Interpretation of typical performance

These vigintiles are used to interpret the median and the interquartile range. Figure 9.1 shows that the player's median values the percentage of points where the first serve is in, the percentage of second serve points that are won, the percentage of receiving points that are break points and the percentage of points where the player hits winners are above average for the relevant population of performances. Specifically, the player's median values for these variables are in the top 40% of values for this level of tennis. By contrast, the player's percentage of double faults played, percentage of break points won and percentage of points where unforced errors are made are relatively low for the given level of tennis. Specifically, the player's median values for these variables are in the lowest 40% of values for the given population of tennis performances. This is actually a good thing in the case of unforced errors and also for double faults, where lower values are preferable. The player's break points performances need to consider the number of break points earned as well as the percentage of these that are converted. The below average conversion rate might not be a problem due to the above average number of break points generated. Similarly, a player's double faults may need to be related to the number of aces played. When these variables are expressed in relative terms in Figure 9.1, we can justify the percentage double faults because reducing this might also reduce the number of aces if the player uses a less risky service strategy.

Interpreting variability in performance

Figure 9.1 also helps us interpret the consistency of the player's performances by looking at the interquartile range in real terms considering the relevant population of tennis performances. The player's most consistent variables are the percentage of break points that are won, the percentage of points won when a second serve is needed, and the percentage of service points that are aces. The player's interquartile ranges for these three variables span 15%,

20% and 25% of all performances at the relevant level of tennis, respectively. The percentage of serving points that are aces is consistently average, being roughly equivalent to the middle 20% of performances for the relevant population of performances. The percentage of points won when a second serve is required is consistently above average, with the interquartile range of the player's performances roughly spanning the fourth quintile of performance in the relevant population (60%–80%). The percentage of break points converted is consistently below average, with the interquartile range of the players performances being located in the bottom half of all performances for this level of tennis. The variable where the player is most inconsistent is the percentage of points won when receiving serve. The player's interquartile range for this variable spans 60% of the relevant population of performances. This is high when one considers that the interquartile range for the relevant population reflects performances from different players with different tactical styles. Figure 9.1 also shows that the player's performances are inconsistent for the percentage of points won when the player goes to the net and the percentage of receiving points that are break points.

Absolute and relative performance

Figure 9.1 makes a slight improvement to the profiling technique as presented in O'Donoghue's (2005) paper. This is the presentation of median values for the performance indicators in parentheses. It is important to include these to avoid confusion between absolute and relative values for performance indicators. For example, consider the 4.1% of service points where the player serves an ace. This is located in the 10th of the 20 bandings between the 45% and 50% percentiles. Without the absolute value presented in parentheses, a reader might think that 47.5% of the player's service points are aces. This would be a misinterpretation of the radar chart which shows the performance indicators in relative terms; the percentage of the relevant population of performances that are exceeded by the player's performances. So, the player does not serve double faults in 25% to 30% of the player's service points either. Realistically, it is more likely that such confusion could occur for other variables such as the percentage of points where the first serve is in, the percentage of points won on first serve and the percentage of points won when a second serve is required.

Profiles of single performances

Opposition quality effect

The profiling technique illustrated in Figure 9.1 is suitable for looking at a set of performances to determine a typical performance and describe the variability about the typical performance. When interpreting the variability in performance, it is worth noting that the performances will have come against opponents of different ability and tactical styles. For example, the profile of the fictitious player shown in Figure 9.1 includes matches from early rounds as well as matches in later rounds such as the quarter-finals and semi-finals. It is reasonable to expect that the percentage of points won on first serve, second serve, when receiving, break points and at the net would be lower against a quarter-finalist or semi-finalist than against an opponent in the early rounds.

Opposition effect leads to potential misinterpretation of performance if O'Donoghue's (2005) technique were to be used with a single performance. The use of norms from the population of relevant performances does not help here. Where a player faces high quality opposition, they would be expected to produce a low value for a performance indicator like the percentage of points won when the first serve is in. This low absolute value for the performance indicator will simply map onto a low 5% banding of values from the relevant population. Similarly, a high value for such a performance indicator achieved against a lower ability opponent will map onto a higher 5% banding. Therefore, O'Donoghue's (2005) technique is not recommended for individual performances because it does not address the effect of opposition quality.

Relative quality

A player's or team's performance in a match not only depends on the quality of the opposition but also on the quality of the player or team themselves. This difference between the quality of the performer and the opponent is referred to as relative quality. In order to determine relative quality, we need a variable to represent player or team quality. This could be a ranking or ranking points, such world rankings and ranking points used in soccer, rugby union and tennis. Consider our fictitious tennis player competing and the opponents faced at the tennis tournament. The opponents' have world rankings and world ranking points that change regularly. Therefore, their rankings or ranking points could be used to represent the quality of the player. A problem with using world rankings is that the same difference between rankings represents a larger gap between higher ranked players than lower ranked players. For example, the world's 101st and 110th ranked players are expected to be more similar in quality that the world's 1st and 10th ranked players. Ranking points, and prize money, can be skewed variables where the top ten players in some sports may win so much money that only the top ten players have an above average prize money within the world's top 100. Klaasen and Magnus (2001) transformed players' world rankings to roughly represent the round of the tournament a player would be expected to get to. For example, players ranked 128th, 64th and 32nd would be expected to reach the first, second and third rounds, respectively. The players ranked 4th and 2nd would be expected to reach the semi-final (which we can think of as round 6) and the final (which we can think of as round 7). This means that we need to use the number 8 to represent the expectation that the top ranked player would not only reach the final, but go one step further and win it. Equation (9.1) shows how Klaasen and Magnus (2001) represent player quality, Q, given their world ranking, R.

$$Q = 8 - \log_2 R \quad (9.1)$$

This means that the relative quality for the top ranked player against the world's number 128 would be +7, given that the top ranked player is expected to get 7 rounds further than the opponent. Similarly, the relative quality for the world's number 512 playing against the world number 1 is −9, because the world number 512 is expected to be eliminated 9 rounds before the world number 1. Basically, the world number 512 would be expected to reach the penultimate qualifying round and be eliminated at that point. Performance indicators for the full population can be correlated (using Pearson's r) with relative quality to determine if there is a relationship. If the coefficient of determination (r^2) is high enough, then a regression equation can be used to determine expected values for performance indicators given the relative quality between the players in a match. A coefficient of determination that is greater than 0.1 means that more than 10% of the performance indicator value is explained by the relative quality of the players. This 10% does not sound like much but does allow us to calculate an expected value for the performance indicator based on the players' world rankings. This is done using regression equations (Cullinane and O'Donoghue, 2011) which have a constant (intercept) and a gradient (slope). The difference between a player's value for the performance indicator and the predicted value can be used to evaluate the performance.

Before moving on to discuss how relative quality can be addressed, it is worth considering what to do about variables with low correlations with relative quality. The relationships between the performance indicators and relative quality do not consider that some players perform better on some court surfaces than others or that some players may have played longer matches earlier in the tournament. Some variables may have no correlation with relative quality. For example, how often the first serve is in is not as important to success as winning points whether on first serve, second serve or when receiving. The percentage of points where a player goes to the net is a tactical variable representing style of play. There may be players who go to the net more than others as well as "baseliners" in all regions of the world rankings. A further issue is that the relationships between relative quality and some performance indicators may be curvilinear rather than linear.

Addressing opposition quality

When comparing two performances, the quality of the player and the opponents is estimated using equation (9.1). These can be used to determine expected values for any performance indicators that are sufficiently correlated with relative quality. The expected value is determined by applying regression equations for these variables to the relative quality between the player and each opponent. Consider two matches, one against an opponent ranked 100th in the World and the other against an opponent ranked 5th. The player wins 64% and 62% of points when the first serve is in during these two matches. It is most likely that the difference between the expected values would be much greater than 1%. Therefore, although the performance against the opponent ranked 5th in the World has a lower value for the percentage of points won when the first serve is in, this may be a better performance in relative terms. For example, the player may have been expected to achieve values of 68% and 60% in these two matches, respectively. Thus, the player will have done better than expected against the opponent ranked 5th in the world and worse than expected against the opponent ranked 100th in the World.

Issues with single match profiles addressing opposition quality

A radar chart presenting a profile for a single match could plot the observed and expected values for each performance indicator to allow areas of better and worse performance than expected to be visually recognised. This does, however, present some issues. If we plot the percentile of the population the observed and expected values exceed (as in Figure 9.1), we may miss subtle differences where the observed and expected values fall within the same 5% band. If, on the other hand, we were to plot the observed and expected values of the performance indicators rather than the 5% band, then we create confusion in that the radar chart for typical performance plots percentage of the population that the player has greater values than but the radar chart for a single match plots performance indicator values. A further issue with plotting actual values on the radar chart is that some values, like aces and double faults, have much lower values than other performance indicators even when expressed as percentages of service points. This problem is worse in profiles from other sports where some of the performance indicators may not be percentages.

Alternative ways of addressing opposition quality

An alternative to using regression-based approaches to addressing opposition quality is to use separate norms for different types of match. For example, British Super League netball teams have been classed as Top Half or Bottom Half (O'Donoghue et al., 2008). This means there are four types of performance; Top Half v Top Half, Top Half v Bottom Half, Bottom Half v Top Half, and Bottom Half v Bottom Half. This approach is only valid where the teams in the top half are very similar in quality and the teams in the bottom half are also similar to each other in terms of quality. A disadvantage of this approach is that it only works where teams within a given half of the league are similar, and a match against one team in a given half of the league is similar to any other in terms of opposition quality. This was the case for one particular season of the British Super League in netball, but usually teams within leagues exhibit more of a gradual increase in quality from bottom to top (Cullinane and O'Donoghue, 2011). A further issue with using separate norms for different types of matches is that the data we use to create the norms is potentially split into multiple subgroups. If we assume 4 qualities of team, we need 16 (4^2) sets of norms for the different types of match. This is because we need norms for each type of team against each type of opponent. This rarely results in the data used to determine norms being split into equal sized subsets. When considering a tournament like the US Open tennis tournament, there may be fewer matches between low ranked players and low ranked opponents because many such players may be eliminated in the 1st round.

A further approach is not to use a quality indicator at all. Instead, we may be able to gather enough evidence to show what is normal against individual teams. An example of this is the work of Nisotaki (2016) that is described in Jayal et al. (2018: 44–48). Nisotaki (2016) found very low correlations between most variables in English FA Premier League soccer and measures of quality such as final league position or final league points. Team games are complex with some teams' success being due to their attack, some teams' success being more to do with their defence, some teams' success due to their creating scoring opportunities and other teams' success being due to their converting opportunities into scores. The relative contribution of tackling, passing, shooting, aerial play, set pieces, goal keeping, etc. form a complex mix of performance areas such that the individual areas in isolation may have low correlations with outcome. This allows areas of strength for individual teams to be recognised. For example, Aston Villa in the 2013–14 season were the 3rd most successful team at defending against opposition passes in their own half, despite finishing the season in 15th place. So what Nisotaki (2016) did was produce separate norms for matches against different teams. The example presented in Jayal et al.'s (2018) book used the percentage of passes in the opposition half that were successful. Each team plays 38 league matches per season allowing quintile norms to be produced for matches against each team. This allows performances against each team to be grouped into 20% bandings for the variable. The advantage of this approach over a regression-based approach is that opponents can be represented by their specific strengths and weaknesses. It may be easier to pass the ball in the opposition half against some teams than against others, and this may be unrelated to the overall quality of the team. These norms not only represent the strength of the team in a particular area of the game but also the consistency of the team in this area. For example, Everton in the 2013–14 season were shown to be more consistent in defending against opposition passing in their own half than Crystal Palace.

Developments in performance profiles

Including opposition performance

The profile for our fictitious tennis player in Figure 9.1 plots the performance indicators in relative terms; the percentage of performances at the given level that the player's value for the performance indicator exceeds. This is done for the average match (median values) and also representing the interquartile range in the performance in relative terms. Players' performances are influenced by the quality and type of opposition they face (O'Donoghue, 2009). Therefore, the performances of the opponents may be influenced by the player's ability to return serve. The performances of the opponents at the net and even how often they decide to come to the net may be influenced by the player's ability to play passing shots and lobs against opponents at the net. The opponents may also come to the net less than the average player in the tournament if the player plays shots that make it difficult for the opponents to play approach shots. Therefore, Figure 9.2 is a profile that includes the values for the opponents on the right-hand side of the radar chart. This chart is not as clear as Figure 9.1 due to the number of variables included. An alternative would be to have six lines in a radar chart like Figure 9.1 instead of three lines; the three additional lines being for the opponents' median, lower and upper quartiles. However, this would be too cluttered. A version

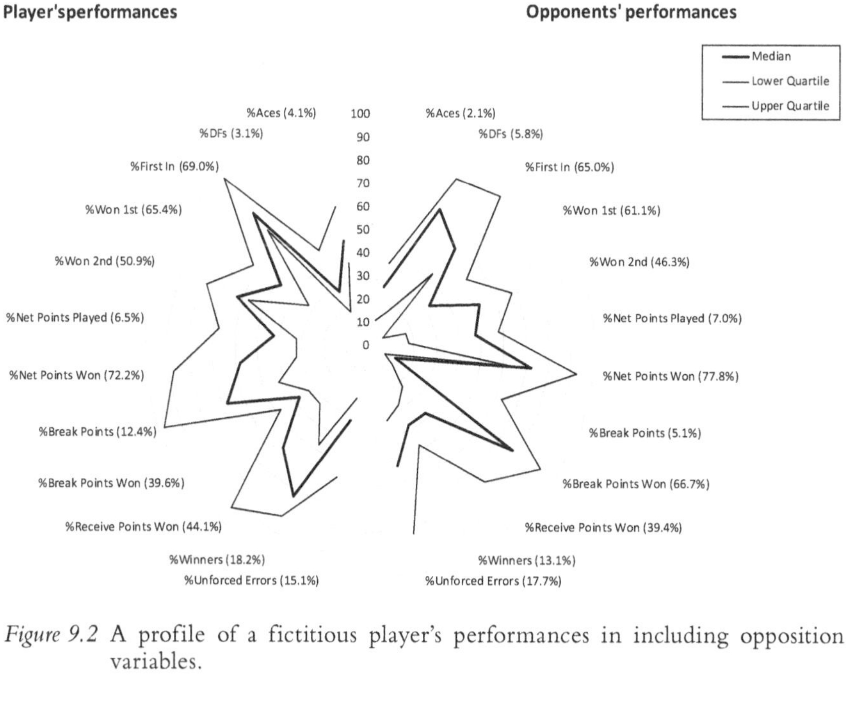

Figure 9.2 A profile of a fictitious player's performances in including opposition variables.

of Figure 9.1 with just the medians for the player and the average opponent would allow a direct comparison between their average performances but would not represent variability in performance.

Therefore, Figure 9.3 uses a line graph instead of a radar chart to represent the performances of the player and the opponents. The second difference to the presentation in Figure 9.3 and Figures 9.1 and 9.2 is that Figure 9.3 uses actual values for the performance indicators rather than the percentage of performances at this level of tennis that the player's and opponents' values exceed. Technically, the variables for points won when receiving serve become redundant in this profile when we have the variables for the opponent's serving performance included. The following observations can be made about the player's performances by considering the opposition values shown in Figure 9.3. Firstly, the player serves more aces and fewer double faults than the opponents. Secondly, the player is consistently winning more points on both first and second serve than the opponents. On both first and second serves, the player's lower quartile for percentage of points won is greater than the upper quartile for the opponents. Thirdly, the average opponent converts a greater percentage of break points than the player does, which may initially seem concerning. However, this needs to be considered along with the number of break points earned and played. Consider the upper quartile for the percentage of break points won by the opponent (100%). This could be because of three matches where the opponents each had one break point which they converted. Fourthly, the final observation is that the player hits

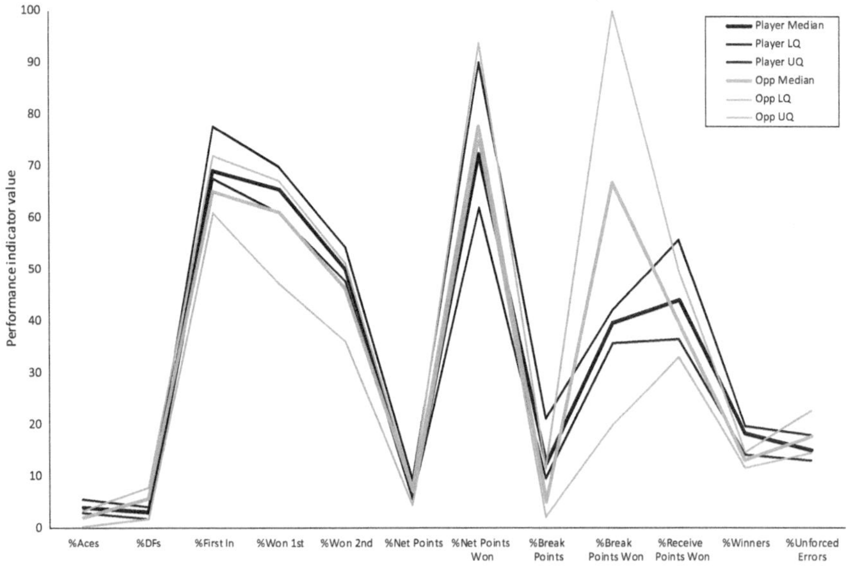

Figure 9.3 A profile presented as a line graph.

more winners and plays fewer unforced errors than the opponents. However, there is some overlap in the interquartile ranges for unforced errors.

Interactive profiles

An interactive profile is dynamic and can change as the user interacts with it, allowing different options to be chosen about what the user wishes to see. Consider the profile shown in Figure 9.3 except shown for individual matches so there are only two lines. The graph can be turned into an interactive dynamic graph through a combination of the VLOOKUP function and "Developer" features in Microsoft Excel. Where we have all data performance indicators for all performances, we can use two cells to hold the name of the player and opponent we are interested in. These names can then be looked up in a performance indicator table where we have a row for each performance, a column for the player, a column for the opponent and a column for each performance indicator. The trick is to have a column representing both players joined together as a single string. This then gives a unique identifying field for each performance. VLOOKUP will look for the combined player names or identities in the left-most column of the performance indicator table. The column being looked up will differ for each performance indicator and be included in the VLOOKUP function for each performance indicator. Thus, when we change the player and opponent of interest, the values that are looked up are changed and any chart that uses these cells will also change when we change the player and opponent of interest.

The analyst can use developer facilities in Microsoft Excel instead of having to type in the player and opponent name. For example, they could use spinner tools, menus or drop-down boxes. Typically, we do not see the "Developer" tab in Microsoft Excel and need to access it. This is done by right clicking on the menu ribbon at the top. A form appears where we can tick that we wish to use the developer tab. Once this is available, we can enter scroll-bars, spinner tools, combo-boxes, etc. into our spreadsheet. These facilities can be used to change the player or opponent we wish to look at.

Multimedia profiles

The main profiling techniques developed by O'Donoghue (2005) and James et al. (2005) present exclusively quantitative performance indicators. Returning to the meanings of the word "profile" listed in the Cambridge Dictionary (2022), it is worth considering the first meaning listed when "profile" is used as a verb; "to write or publish a short description of someone's life, work, character, etc.". If I were to tell you that there was going to be a profile of Lionel Messi on television this evening, what would you expect the programme to be like? It would probably be a documentary that includes facts, figures, video sequences, interviews, pictures and charts. This has motivated the development of multimedia performance profiles to go beyond quantitative data and incorporate other forms of information in profiles (Butterworth, 2017; 2023c). These profiles present quantitative performance indicators as before highlighting areas of good, not so good, average, consistent and inconsistent performance as previous techniques have done. However, multimedia performance profiles are made dynamic with supporting clips illustrating quality of play, tactics used and consistency of play. The research implemented multimedia profiles for badminton and netball and was implemented in Prezi (Prezi Inc., San Francisco, Ca). It is true that commercial video analysis packages allow video sequences of events satisfying criteria of interest to be presented with great flexibility within the packages. However, this does not work so well for typical profiles based on multiple matches. Hence, the development of multimedia profiles by Butterworth (2017, 2023c) to go beyond the profiling techniques of O'Donoghue (2005) and James et al. (2005).

Conclusions

Profiling in sports performance analysis, like profiling in other areas of sports science, involves bringing together different variables to for a profile. The variables should be valid and reliable and preferably possess the qualities for being performance indicators. Variables in sports performance differ from variables in other areas of sports science in that they can be highly inconsistent between matches, mainly because of varying opposition effects. Therefore, profiles in sports performance analysis need to represent the level of consistency or inconsistency in performance as well as the typical (average performance). Advances in technology allow greater flexibility in presenting performance profiles and recent developments have also introduced multimedia data into profiles.

References

Aksum, K.M., Brotangen, L., Bjørndal, C.T., Magnaguagno, L., & Jordet, G. (2021) 'Scanning activity of elite football players in 11 vs 11 match play: an eye-tracking analysis on the duration and visual information of scanning', *PLOS ONE*, 16(8): e0244118. DOI: 10.1371/journal.pone.0244118

Altman, D.G. (1991) *Practical statistics for medical research*, London: Chapman & Hall.

Andersen, L.W., Francis, J.W., & Bateman, M. (2022) 'Danish association football coaches' perception of performance analysis', *International Journal of Performance Analysis in Sport*, 22(1): 149–173. DOI: 10.1080/24748668.2021.2012040

APFA (n.d.), Twitter account of the Association of Professional Football Analysts, https://twitter.com/APFAnalysis, accessed 20th July 2023.

Araujo, D., Davids, K., & Hristovski, R. (2006) 'The ecological dynamics of decision making in sport', *Psychology of Sport Exercise*, 7(6): 653–676.

Ashford, M., Taylor, J., Payne, J., Waldouck, D., & Collins, D. (2023) 'Getting on the same page: enhancing team performance with shared mental models: case studies of evidence informed practice in elite sport', *Frontiers in Sports and Active Living*, 5, 1057143. DOI: 10.3389/fspor.2023.1057143

Barreira, D., Garganta, J., Machado, J., & Anguera, M.T (2014) 'Effects of ball recovery on top-level soccer attacking patterns of play', *Revista brasileira de cineantropometria & desempenho humano*, 16(1): 36–46. DOI: 10.5007/1980-0037.2014v16n1p36

BASES (2023) British Association of Sport and Exercise Sciences 2023: abstract submissions, https://www.delegate-reg.co.uk/bases2023/submissions, accessed 9th August 2023.

Bateman, M., & Jones, G. (2019) 'Strategies for maintaining the coach-analyst relationship within professional football utilizing the COMPASS model: the performance analyst's perspective', *Frontiers in Psychology*, 10. DOI: 10.3389/fpsyg.2019.02064

Benton, T.R., Ross, D.F., Bradshaw, E., Thomas, W.N., & Bradshaw, G.S. (2006) 'Eyewitness memory is still not common sense', *Applied Cognitive Psychology*, 20, 115–129. DOI: 10.1002/acp.1171

Bester, C., Coetzee, D., Schall, R., & Blair, M. (2019) 'Physical demands on elite lead rugby union referees', *International Journal of Performance Analysis in Sport*, 19(2): 258–273. DOI: 10.1080/24748668.2019.1593097

Bevan, N. (1995) 'Measuring usability as quality of use', *Software Quality Journal*, 4: 115–130.

Blair, M.R., Scanlan, A.T., Lastella, M., Ramsey, C., & Elsworthy, N. (2022) 'The relationships between physical fitness attributes and match demands in rugby union referees officiating the 2019 Rugby World Cup', *International Journal of Performance Analysis in Sport*, 22(1): 183–194. DOI: 10.1080/24748668.2022.2031527

Bliss, A., Ahmun, R., Jowitt, H., Scott, P., Callaghan, S., Jones, T.W., & Tallent, J. (2022) 'Variability of test match cricket and the effects of match location on physical demands in male seam bowlers', *International Journal of Performance Analysis in Sport*, 22(2): 291–301. DOI: 10.1080/24748668.2022.2051924

Bloomfield, J., Polman, R., & O'Donoghue, P. (2004) 'The Bloomfield movement classification: motion analysis of individual players in dynamic movement sports', *International Journal of Performance Analysis in Sport*, 4(2): 20–31. DOI: 10.1080/24748668.2004.11868300

Bogen, E.M., Schlachta, C., & Ponsky, T. (2019) 'White paper: technology for surgical telemento- ring-SAGES Project 6 Technology Working Group', *Surgical Endoscopy*, 33: 684–690. DOI: 10.1002/jso.26524

Bornstein, B. (2017) *Popular myths about memory*, New York: Lexington Books.

Bracewell, P.J., Meyer, D., & Ganesh, S. (2003) 'Creating and monitoring meaningful individual rugby ratings', *Research Letters in the Information and Mathematical Sciences*, 4: 19–22.

Bradley, P.S. (2020) Football decoded: using match analysis and context to interpret the demands, Independently published, ISBN: 979-8572156942.

Briki, W., Hartigh, R.J.D., Bakker, C.F., & Gernigon, C. (2012) 'The dynamics of psychological momentum: a quantitative study in natural sport situations', *International Journal of Performance Analysis in Sport*, 12(3): 573–592. DOI: 10.1080/24748668.2012.11868620

Brown, E., & O'Donoghue, P.G. (2008) 'A split screen system to analyse coach behaviour: a case report of coaching practice', *International Journal of Computer Science in Sport*, 7(1): 4–17.

Bruce, L., Farrow, D., Raynor, A., & May, E. (2009) 'Notation analysis of skill expertise differences in netball', *International Journal of Performance Analysis in Sport*, 9(2): 245–254. DOI: 10.1080/24748668.2009.11868481

Bučar, M., Čuk, I., Pajek, J., Karacsony, I., & Leskošek, B. (2012) 'Reliability and validity of judging in women's artistic gymnastics at University Games 2009', *European Journal of Sport Science*, 12(3): 207–215. DOI: 10.1080/17461391.2010.551416

Budrionis, A., Bellika, J.G., Augestad, K.M., & Patel, H.R.H. (2013) 'An evaluation framework for defining the contributions of telestration in surgical telementoring', *Journal of Medical Internet Research*, 15(7): 14. DOI: 10.2196/ijmr.2611

Budrionis, A., Hasvold, P., Hartvigsen, G., & Bellika, J.G. (2015) 'Assessing the impact of telestration on surgical telementoring: a randomized controlled trial', *Journal of Telemedicine and Telecare*, 22(1): 12–17. DOI: 10.1177/1357633X15585071

Brümmer, K (2019) 'Coordination in sports teams: ethnographic insights into practices of video analysis in football', *European Journal for Sport and Society*, 16(1): 27–43. DOI: 10.1080/16138171.2019.1603682

Butler, R.J., & Hardy, L. (1992) 'The performance profile: theory and application', *Sport Psychologist*, 6: 253–264.

Butler, R.J. (1996) *Performance profiling*, Leeds: National Coaching Foundation.

Butterworth, A. (2017) 'Multimedia performance profiles', Ph.D Thesis, Cardiff, UK: Cardiff Metropolitan University.

Butterworth, A. (2023a) 'Emerging technology and interactive feedback', In A. Butterworth (ed.), *Professional practice in sport performance analysis* (pp. 19–46). London: Routledge.

Butterworth, A. (2023b) 'Performance analysis in an interdisciplinary sports science team', In A. Butterworth (ed.), *Professional practice in sport performance analysis* (pp. 47–62). London: Routledge.

Butterworth, A. (2023c) 'Multimedia performance profiling', In A. Butterworth (ed.), *Professional practice in sport performance analysis* (pp. 63–88). London: Routledge.

Butterworth, A. (2023d) 'Career development and professional literacy', In A. Butterworth (ed.), *Professional practice in sports performance analysis* (pp. 133–149). London: Routledge.

Butterworth, A., & O'Donoghue, P.G. (2023) 'Health, safety and ethics for the professional practitioner', In A. Butterworth (ed.), *Professional practice in sports performance analysis* (pp. 150–165). London: Routledge.

Butterworth, A.D., Turner, D.J., & Johnstone, J.A. (2012) 'Coaches' perceptions of the potential use of performance analysis in badminton', *International Journal of Performance Analysis in Sport*, 12(2): 452–467. DOI:10.1080/24748668.2012.11868610

Cambridge Dictionary (2022) 'profile', https://dictionary.cambridge.org/dictionary/english/profile, accessed 29th January 2022.

Carling, C., Williams, M.A., & Reilly, T. (2005) *Handbook of soccer match analysis: a systematic approach to improving performance*, London & New York: Routledge.

Cassidy, T., Jones, R.L., & Potrac, P. (2009) *Understanding sports coaching: the social, cultural and pedagogical foundations of coaching practice*, 2nd edition, Oxon: Routledge.

Catapult (2023) Catapult: Basketball performance solutions, https://www.catapult.com/sports/basketball, accessed 16th August 2023.

CDC (2022) 'About child and teen BMI', https://www.cdc.gov/healthyweight/assessing/bmi/childrens_bmi/about_childrens_bmi.html, accessed 27th July 2023.

Coach Logic (2023) Streamline your video analysis, https://www.coach-logic.com, accessed 16th August 2023.

Cohen, J. (1960) 'A coefficient of agreement for nominal scales', *Educational and Psychological Measurement*, 20: 37–46. DOI: 10.1177/001316446002000104

Cohen, J. (1968) 'Weighted kappa: nominal scale agreement with provision for scaled agreement or partial credit', *Psychological Bulletin*, 70: 213–220. DOI: 10.1037/h0026256

Cooper, D., & Pulling, C. (2020) 'The impact of ball recovery type, location of ball recovery and duration of possession on the outcomes of possessions in the English Premier League and the Spanish La Liga', *Science and Medicine in Football*, 4(3): 196–202. DOI: 10.1080/24733938.2020.1722319

Coves, A., Caballero, C., & Moreno, F.J. (2020) 'Relationship between kinematic variability and performance in basketball free-throw', *International Journal of Performance Analysis in Sport*, 20(6): 931–941. DOI: 10.1080/24748668.2020.1820172.

Cuevas, C., Quilón, D., & García, N. (2020) 'Techniques and applications for soccer video analysis: a survey', *Multimedia Tools and Applications*, 79(39–40): 29685–29721.

Cullinane, A., & O'Donoghue, P.G. (2011) 'Addressing opposition quality in rugby league performance', poster presented at the World Congress of Science and Football, Nagoya, Japan, May 2011.

Cunniffe, E., Connor, M., Beato, M., Grainger, A., McConnell, W., McCarthy Persson, Ulrik., Delahunt, E., Boreham, C., & Blake, C. (2022) 'The influence of possession status on the physical output of male international hockey players', *International Journal of Sports Science and Coaching*, 17(2): 412–422. DOI: 10.1177/174795412110339

Cushion, C. (2018) 'Observing coach behaviours: developing coaching practice and coach education', In R. Thelwell, & M. Dicks (eds.), *Professional advances in sports coaching* (pp. 358–376). London: Routledge.

Dartfish (n.d.-a) https://www.youtube.com/watch?v=wZBOJnJM1XA, accessed 5th August 2023.

Dartfish (n.d.-b) https://www.youtube.com/watch?v=8ctkzUqoYtk, accessed 5th August 2023.

Datavolley (2022) 'Scout and analyse your match', https://www.dataproject.com/Products/US/en/Volleyball/DataVolley, accessed 29th January 2022.

Dellal, A., Lago-Peñas, C., Rey, E., Chamari, K., & Orhant, E. (2015) 'The effects of a congested fixture period on physical performance, technical activity and injury rate during matches in a professional soccer team', *British Journal of Sports Medicine*, 49(6): 390–394. DOI: 10.1007/s40279-020-01359-9

Dos Reis, M.A.M., & Almeida, M.B. (2020) 'The role of somatic maturation in the tactical effectiveness, efficiency and variability of young soccer players', *International Journal of Performance Analysis in Sport*, 20(2): 305–321. DOI: 10.1080/24748668.2020.1743165

Dickersin, K., Min, Y.I., & Meinert, C.L. (1992) 'Factors influencing publication of research results: follow-up of applications submitted to two institutional review boards', *Journal of the American Medical Association*, 267(3): 374–378. PMID: 1727960.

Dinnie, A., & O'Donoghue, P.G. (2020) 'Strategic target setting in the heptathlon', *Journal of Sports Analytics*, 6(2): 129–145. DOI: 10.3233/JSA-200351

Drust, B. (2010) 'Performance analysis research: meeting the challenge', *Journal of Sports Sciences*, 28(9): 921–922. DOI: 10.1080/02640411003740769

EIS (2021) 'Performance Support', https://eis2win.co.uk/service/performance-support/, accessed 29th January 2022.

Engeness, I., & Lund, A. (2020) 'Learning for the future: Insights arising from the contributions of Piotr Galperin to the cultural-historical theory', *Learning, Culture and Social Interaction*, 25: 100257. DOI: 10.1016/j.lcsi.2018.11.004

ESPN (2022) 'Cricinfo', https://www.espncricinfo.com/, accessed 29th January 2022.

Fele, G., & Campagnolo, G.M. (2021) 'Expertise and the work of football match analysts in TV sport broadcasts', *Discourse studies*, 23(5): 616–635: 10.1177/14614456211016799

Fernandez-Echeverria, C., Mesquita, I., Conejero, M., & Moreno, M.P. (2019) 'Perceptions of elite volleyball players on the importance of match analysis during the training process', International Journal of Performance Analysis in Sport, 19(1): 49–64. DOI: 10.1080/24748668.2018.1559544

FIFA (n.d.) 'Study the FIFA Football Language', https://www.fifatrainingcentre.com/en/resources-tools/football-language/, accessed 10th August 2023.

FIFA (2023) FIFA Metrics - Final third entries. https://www.fifatrainingcentre.com, accessed 13th August 2023.

Fischer, M.T., Keim, D.A., & Stein, M. (2019) 'Video-based analysis of soccer matches', Proceedings of the 2nd International Workshop on Multimedia Content Analysis in Sports (MMSports '19), 1–9.

Flick, H. (2016) 'Use of performance analysis by the German men's national soccer squad', invited seminar, 6th International Teaching Games for Understanding conference, Cologne, Germany.

Flightscope (nodate) https://flightscope.com, accessed 28th July 2023.

Francis, J., & Jones, G. (2014) 'Elite rugby union players perceptions of performance analysis', *International Journal of Performance Analysis in Sport*, 14(1): 188–207. DOI: 10.1080/24748668.2014.11868714

Franks, I.M. (1997) 'Use of feedback by coaches and players', In T. Reilly, J. Bangsbo, & M. Hughes (eds.), *Science and Football 3* (pp. 267–278). London: E and FN Spon.

Franks, I.M., & Miller, G. (1986) 'Eyewitness testimony in sport', *Journal of Sport Behavior*, 9(1): 38–45.

Franks, I.M., & Miller, G. (1991) 'Training coaches to observe and remember', *Journal of Sports Science*, 9(3): 285–297. DOI: 10.1080/02640419108729890

Franks, I.M., Hodges, N., & More, K. (2001) 'Analysis of coaching behaviour', *International Journal of Performance Analysis in Sport*, 1(1): 27–36. DOI: 10.1080/24748668.2001.11868246

French, J., & Raven, B. (1959) 'The bases of social power', In D. Cartwright (ed.), *Studies in Social Power* (pp. 150–167), Ann Arbor, MI: Institute for Social Research.

Furley, P., Moll, T., & Memmert, D. (2015) 'Put your hands up in the air? The interpersonal effects of pride and shame expressions on opponents and teammates', *Frontiers of Psychology*, 6: 1361. DOI: 10.3389/fpsyg.2015.01361

Galily, Y. (2014) 'When the medium becomes "well done": sport, television, and technology in the twenty-first century', *Television & New Media*, 15(8): 717–724. DOI: 10.1177/1527476414532141

Gangstead, S.K., & Beveridge, S.K. (1984) 'The implementation and evaluation of a methodical approach to qualitative sport skill analysis instruction', *Journal of Teaching in Physical Education*, 3, 60–70. DOI: 10.1123/jtpe.3.2.60

García-Marín, P., & Iturriaga, F.M.A. (2017) 'Water polo: technical and tactical shot indicators between winners and losers according to the final score of the game', *International Journal of Performance Analysis in Sport*, 17(3): 334–349. DOI: 10.1080/24748668.2017.1339258

García-Santos, D., Gómez-Ruano, M-Á., Vaquera, A., & Ibáñez, S.J. (2020) 'Systematic review of basketball referees' performances', *International Journal of Performance Analysis in Sport*, 20(3): 495–533. DOI: 10.1080/24748668.2020.1758437

Gerisch, G., & Reichelt, M. (1993) 'Computer and video aided analysis of football games', In T. Reilly, J. Clarys, & A. Stibbe (eds.), *Science and Football II* (pp. 167–174). London: E & FN Spon.

Gibbs, G. (1988) *Learning by doing: a guide to teaching and learning methods*, Oxford: Oxford Further Education Unit.

Gómez, M- Á., Lago-Peñas, C., & Pollard, R. (2013) 'Situational variables', In T. McGarry, P.G. O'Donoghue, & J. Sampaio (eds.), *Routledge handbook of sports performance analysis* (pp. 259–269). London: Routledge.

Gong, B., Cui, Y., Zhang, S., Zhou, C., Yi, Q., & Gómez-Ruano, M-Á (2021) 'Impact of technical and physical key performance indicators on ball possession in the Chinese Super League', *International Journal of Performance Analysis in Sport*, 21(6): 909–921. DOI: 10.1080/24748668.2021.1957296

Gregson, W., Drust, B., Atkinson, G., & Salvo, V.D. (2010) 'Match-to-match variability of high-speed activities in premier league soccer', *International Journal of Sports Medicine*, 31(4): 237–242. DOI: 10.1055/s-0030-1247546

Groom, R., & Cushion, C. (2005) 'Using of video based coaching with players: a case study', *International Journal of Performance Analysis in Sport*, 5(3): 40–46: DOI: 10.1080/24748668.2005.11868336

Groom, R., & Nelson, L. (2013) 'The application of video-based performance analysis: the coach supporting athlete learning', In: P. Potrac, W. Gilbert, & J. Denison, (eds.), *Routledge Handbook of Sports Coaching* (pp. 96–107). Oxon: Routledge.

Groom, R., Cushion, C., & Nelson, L. (2011) 'The delivery of video-based performance analysis by England youth soccer coaches: towards a grounded theory', *Journal of Applied Sport Psychology*, 23(1): 16–32. DOI: 10.1080/10413200.2010.511422

Groom, R., Cushion, C.J., & Nelson, L.J. (2012) 'Analysing coach-athlete "talk in interaction" within the delivery of video-based performance feedback in elite youth soccer', *Qualitative Research in Sport, Exercise and Health*, 4(3): 439–458. DOI: 10.1080/2159676X.2012.693525

Gucciardi, D.F., & Gordon, S. (2009) 'Revisiting the performance profile technique: theoretical underpinnings and application', *The Sport Psychologist*, 23: 93–117. DOI: 10.1123/tsp.23.1.93

Hawk-eye (n.d.) http://www.hawkeyeinnovations.co.uk/page/sports-officiating/tennis, accessed 29th July 2013.

Hay, J.G. (1988) 'Approach strategies in the long jump', *International Journal of Sports Biomechanics*, 4: 114–129. DOI: 10.1123/ijsb.4.2.114

Hayes, M. (1997) 'When is research not research? When it's notational analysis', *BASES Newsletter*, 7(7): 4–5.

Hogg, J. (2002) 'Debriefing: a means to increasing recovery and subsequent performance', In M. Kellmann (ed.), *Enhancing recovery: Preventing under-performance in athletes* (pp. 181–198). Champaign, IL: Human Kinetics.

Hopkins, W.G., & Hewson, D.J. (2001) 'Variability of competitive performance of distance runners', *Medicine and Science in Sports and Exercise*, 33(9): 1588–1592. DOI: 10.1097/00005768-200109000-00023

Horne, S. (2013) 'The role of performance analysis in elite netball competition structures', In D.M. Peters, & P.G. O'Donoghue (eds.), *Performance Analysis of Sport IX* (pp. 30–37). London: Routledge.

HUDL (2023) 'Change the way you see the game', https://www.hudl.com, accessed 16th August 2023.

Huggan, R., Nelson, L., & Potrac, P. (2015) 'Developing micropolitical literacy in professional soccer: a performance analyst's tale', *Qualitative Research in Sport, Exercise and Health*, 7(4): 504–520. DOI: 10.1080/2159676X.2014.949832

Hughes, M. (1998) 'The application of notational analysis to racket sports', In A. Lees, I. Maynard, M. Hughes, & T. Reilly (eds.), *Science and racket sports 2* (pp. 211–220). London: E & FN Spon.

Hughes, M., & Bartlett, R. (2002) 'The use of performance indicators in performance analysis', *Journal of Sport Sciences*, 20: 739–754. DOI: 10.1080/026404102320675602

Hughes, M., & Franks, I. (2004) 'How to develop a notation system', In M.D. Hughes, & I.M. Franks (eds.), *Notational analysis of sport: systems for better coaching and performance in sport, 2nd edition* (pp. 118–140). London: Routledge.

Hughes, M., & Franks, I. (2005) 'Analysis of passing sequences, shots and goals in soccer', *Journal of Sports Sciences*, 23(5): 509–514. DOI: 10.1080/02640410410001716779

Hughes, M.D., & Franks, I.M. (2008) *The essentials of performance analysis: an introduction*, Oxon: Routledge.

Hughes, M.D., Evans, S., & Wells, J. (2001) 'Establishing normative profiles in performance analysis', *International Journal of Performance Analysis of Sport*, 1(1): 4–27. DOI: 10.1080/24748668.2001.11868245

In-Play Sports (2023) In-Play Online, https://www.in-playsports.com, accessed 16th August 2023.

International Football Association Board (2023) Laws of the game: football laws, rules and regulations, https://www.theifab.com, accessed: 16th August 2023.

Irwin, G., Bezodis, I., & Kerwin, D. (2013) 'Biomechanics for coaches', In R. Jones, & K. Kingston (eds.), *An Introduction to sports coaching: connecting theory to practice, 2nd edition* (pp. 145–160). London: Routledge.

James, N., Mellalieu, S.D., & Jones, N.M.P. (2005) 'The development of position-specific performance indicators in professional rugby union', *Journal of Sports Sciences*, 23: 63–72. DOI: 10.1080/02640410410001730106

Jayal, A., McRobert, A., Oatley, G., & O'Donoghue, P.G. (2018) *Sports analytics: analysis, visualisation and decision making in sports performance*, London: Routledge.

Jennings, D., Cormack, S., Coutts, J., & Aughey, R.J. (2012) 'GPS analysis of an international field hockey tournament', *International Journal of Sports Physiology and Performance*, 7(3): 224–231. DOI: 10.1123/ijspp.7.3.224

Johns, P., & Brouner, J. (2013) 'The efficacy of judging within trampolining', In D.M. Peters, & P.G. O'Donoghue (eds.), *Performance Analysis of Sport IX* (pp. 214–221). London: Routledge.

Jones, D., Rands, S., & Butterworth, A.D. (2020) 'The use and perceived value of telestration tools in elite football', *International Journal of Performance Analysis in Sport*, 20(3): 373–388. DOI: 10.1080/24748668.2020.1753965

Jones, P.D., James, N., & Mellalieu, S.D. (2004) 'Possession as a performance indicator in soccer', *International Journal of Performance Analysis in Sport*, 4, 98–102. DOI: 10.1080/24748668.2004.11868295

Knudson, D.V. (2013) *Qualitative diagnosis of human movement, 3rd edition*, Champaign Il.: Human Kinetics.

Kádár, L., Géczi, G., Bognár, J., & Csáki, I. (2023) 'Movement analysis of match play in U16-U21 youth Hungarian soccer players: the influence of age, position, and contextual variables', *International Journal of Performance Analysis in Sport*, 23(3): 213–231. DOI: 10.1080/24748668.2023.2219490

Kirkbride, T. (2013) 'Media applications of performance analysis', In T. McGarry, P.G. O'Donoghue, & J. Sampaio (eds.), *Routledge handbook of sports performance analysis* (pp. 187–209). London: Routledge.

Klaasen, F.J.G.M., & Magnus, J.R. (2001) 'Are points in tennis independent and identically distributed? Evidence from a dynamic binary panel data model', *Journal of the American Statistical Association*, 96: 500–509. DOI: 10.1198/016214501753168217

Klemp, M., Wunderlich, F., & Memmert, D. (2021) 'In-play forecasting in football using event and positional data', *Scientific Reports*, 11(1): 24139–24139. DOI: 10.1038/s41598-021-03157-3

Kojman, Y., Beeching, K., Gomez, M-Á., Parmar, N., & Nicholls, S.B. (2022) 'The role of debriefing in enhancing learning and development in professional boxing', *International Journal of Performance Analysis in Sport*, 22(2): 250–260. DOI: 10.1080/24748668.2022.2042640

Koo, D.H., Panday, S.B., Xu, D.Y., Lee, C.Y., & Kim, H.Y. (2016) 'Logistic regression of wins and losses in Asia League ice hockey in the 2014-2015 season', *International Journal of Performance Analysis in Sport*, 16(3): 871–880. DOI: 10.1080/24748668.2016.11868935

Kumar, R. (2005) *Research methodology: a step by step guide for beginners*, 2nd edition, London: Sage.

Laborde, C.J., Bell, C.S., Slaughter, J.C., Valdastri, P., & Obstein, K.L. (2017) 'Evaluation of a novel tablet application for improvement in colonoscopy training and mentoring (with video)', *Gastrointestinal Endoscopy*, 85(3): 559–565. DOI: 10.1016/j.gie.2016.07.052

Lacy, A.C., & Darst, P.W. (1989) 'The Arizona State University Observation Instrument (ASUOI)', In P.W. Darst, D.B. Zakrajsek, & V.H. Mancini (eds.), *Analyzing physical education and sport instruction: Second edition* (pp. 369–378). Champaign, IL: Human Kinetics.

Lafont, D. (2008) 'Gaze control during the hitting phase in tennis: a preliminary study', *International Journal of Performance Analysis in Sport*, 8(1): 85–100. DOI: 10.1080/24748668.2008.11868425

Lago, C. (2009) 'The influence of match location, quality of opposition and match status on possession strategies in professional association football', *Journal of Sports Sciences*, 27: 1463–1469. DOI: 10.1080/02640410903131681

Laird, P., & Waters, L. (2008) 'Eyewitness recollection of sport coaches', *International Journal of Performance Analysis in Sport*, 8(1): 76–84. DOI: 10.1080/24748668.2008.11868424

Lames, M. (1994) *Systematische Spielbeobachtung*, Münster, Germany: Philippka.

Laxdal, A., Ivarsson, A., Sigurgeirsson, O., & Haugen, T. (2022) 'Are the playoffs different from the regular season? A comparison of in-game statistics in Icelandic elite handball', *International Journal of Performance Analysis in Sport*, 22(5): 649–655. DOI: 10.1080/24748668.2022.2115781

Lees, A. (2002) 'Technique analysis in sports: a critical review', *Journal of Sports Sciences*, 20(10): 813–828. DOI: 10.1080/026404102320675657

Leite, W. (2020) 'The importance of set plays in high performance football', *Sportske nauke i zdravlje*, 19(1): 5–9. DOI: 10.7251/JIT2001005L

Lemmink, K., & Frencken, W. (2013) 'Tactical performance analysis in invasion games: perspectives from a dynamic system approach with examples from soccer', In T. McGarry, P. O'Donoghue, & J. Sampaio (eds.), *Routledge handbook of sports performance analysis* (pp. 89–100). Oxon: Routledge.

Leser, R., & Roemer, K. (2015) 'Motion tracking and analysis systems', In A. Baca, (ed.), *Computer science in sport: research and practice* (pp. 82–109). London: Routledge.

Lewis, M., McNicholas, E., McCarthy, A-M., & Sherwin, I. (2023) 'Analysis of referee in-game interactions with players and other officials in professional Rugby Union', *International Journal of Performance Analysis in Sport*, 23(3): 232–248. DOI: 10.1080/24748668.2023.2220528

Lima e Silva, L., Neves, E., Silva, J., Alonso, L., Vale, R., & Nunes, R. (2020) 'The haemodynamic demand and the attributes related to the displacement of the soccer referees in the moments of decision / intervention during the matches', *International Journal of Performance Analysis in Sport*, 20(2): 219–230. DOI: 10.1080/24748668.2020.1736937

Liu, W., Zhou, Z., Shen, Y., & Zhang, H. (2022) 'Stroke performance relevance model for elite table tennis matches', *International Journal of Performance Analysis in Sport*, 22(4): 558–570. DOI: 10.1080/24748668.2022.2089514

Loftus, E.F. (2019) 'Eyewitness testimony', *Cognitive Psychology*, 33(4): 498–503. DOI: 10.1002/acp.3542

Loo, J.K., Francis, J.W., & Bateman, M. (2020) 'Athletes' and coaches' perspectives of performance analysis in women's sports in Singapore', *International Journal of Performance Analysis in Sport*, 20(6): 960–981. DOI: 10.1080/24748668.2020.1820174

Lorains, M., Ball, K., & MacMahon, C. (2013) 'Performance analysis for decision making in team sports', *International Journal of Performance Analysis in Sport*, 13(1): 110–119. DOI: 10.1080/24748668.2013.11868635

Luedeker, B., & McGee, M. (2023) 'Relationship between judges' scores and dive attributes from a video recording of a diving competition', *PLoS One*, 17(8): e0273374. DOI: 10.1371/journal.pone.0273374.

Machado, G., González-Víllora, S., Sarmento, H., & Teoldo, I. (2020) 'Development of tactical decision-making skills in youth soccer players: macro- and microstructure of soccer developmental activities as a discriminant of different dkill levels', *International Journal of Performance Analysis in Sport*, 20(6): 1072–1091. DOI: 10.1080/24748668.2020.1829368

Machado, G., González-Víllora, S., & Teoldo, I. (2023) 'Selected soccer players are quicker and better decision-makers in elite Brazilian youth academies', *International Journal of Performance Analysis in Sport*, 23(2): 65 82. DOI: 10.1080/24748668.2023.2181609

Magill, S., Nelson, L., Jones., R., & Potrac, P. (2017) 'Emotions, identity, and power in video-based feedback sessions: tales from women's professional football', *Sports Coaching Review*, 6(2): 216–232. DOI: 10.4324/9781351024501-6

Malcata, R.M., & Hopkins, W.G. (2014) 'Variability of competitive performance of elite athletes: a systematic review', *Sports Medicine*, 44(12): 1763–1774. DOI: 10.1007/s40279-014-0239-x.

Martens, R. (1987) 'Science, knowledge, and sport psychology', *The Sport Psychologist*, 1(1): 46. DOI: 10.1123/tsp.1.1.29

Martens, R., Vealey, R.S., & Burton, D. (1990) *Competitive anxiety in sport*, Champaign, IL: Human Kinetics.

Martin, D., Swanton, A., Bradley, J., & McGrath, D. (2018) 'The use, integration and perceived value of performance analysis to professional and amateur Irish coaches', *International Journal of Sports Science & Coaching*, 13(4): 520–532. DOI: 10.1177/1747954117753806

Martin, D., O Donoghue, P.G., Bradley, J., & McGrath, D. (2021) 'Developing a framework for professional practice in applied performance analysis', *International Journal of Performance Analysis in Sport*, 21(6): 845–888. DOI: 10.1080/24748668.2021.1951490

Maslovat, D., & Franks, I.M. (2020) 'The importance of feedback to performance', In M. Hughes, I.M. Franks, & H. Dancs (eds.), *Essentials of performance analysis in sport: third edition* (pp. 3–10). Oxon: Routledge.

Mason, R.J., Farrow, D., & Hattie, J.A. (2021) 'An exploratory investigation into the reception of verbal and video feedback provided to players in an Australian Football League club', *International Journal of Sports Science & Coaching*, 16(1): 181–191. DOI: 10.1177/1747954120951080

Mateus, N., Gonçalves, B., Abade, E., Liu, H., Torres-Ronda, L., Leite, N., & Sampaio, J. (2015) 'Game-to-game variability of technical and physical performance in NBA players', *International Journal of Performance Analysis in Sport*, 15(3): 764–776. DOI: 10.1080/24748668.2015.11868829

Mayfield, K. (2002) 'Senegal: the computer's choice', https://www.wired.com/2002/06/senegal-the-computers-choice/, accessed 20th July 2023.

McGarry, T., & Franks, I.M. (1994) 'A stochastic approach to predicting competition squash match-play' *Journal of Sports Sciences*, 12: 573–584. DOI: 10.1080/02640419408732208

McIntyre, M.C., & Hall, M. (2005) 'Physiological profile in relation to playing position of elite college Gaelic footballers', *British Journal of Sports Medicine*, 39: 264–266. DOI: 10.1136/bjsm.2003.011254

McKenna, M., Cowan, D.T., Stevenson, D., & Baker, J.S. (2018). Neophyte experiences of football (soccer) match analysis: a multiple case study approach. *Research in Sports Medicine*, 26(3), 306–322. https://doi.org/10.1080/15438627.2018.1447473

McNair, D.M., Lorr, M., & Droppleman, L. (1971) *Manual for the Profile of Mood States*, San Diego, CA: Educational and Industrial Testing Service.

McRobert, A.P., & Williams, A. M. (2019). Integrating performance analysis and perceptual-cognitive training. In Anticipation and Decision Making in Sport (1st ed., pp. 327–341). Routledge. https://doi.org/10.4324/9781315146270-18

Mellalieu, S., Hanton, S., & O'Brien, M. (2004) 'Intensity and direction of competitive anxiety as a function of sport type and experience', *Scandinavian Journal of Medicine and Science in Sport*, 14(5): 326–334. DOI: 10.1111/j.1600-0838.2004.00389.x

Miarka, B., Fukuda, H.D., Heinisch, H-D., Battazza, R., Del Vecchio, F.B., Camey, S., & Franchini, E. (2016) 'Time-motion analysis and decision making in female judo athletes during victory or defeat at Olympic and non-Olympic events: are combat actions really unpredictable?', *International Journal of Performance Analysis in Sport*, 16(2): 442–463. DOI: 10.1080/24748668.2016.11868900

Middlemas, S.G., Croft, H.G., & Watson, F. (2018). Behind closed doors: The role of debriefing and feedback in a professional rugby team. *International Journal of Sports Science & Coaching*, 13(2), 201–212. https://doi.org/10.1177/1747954117739548

Migdalski, A.H., & Stone, J.A. (2019) 'Investigating lineout performance between the top and bottom four English Premiership rugby union teams in the 2016/17 season', *International Journal of Performance Analysis in Sport*, 19(1): 131–141. DOI: 10.1080/24748668.2019.1570459

Morgan, K., Mouchet, A., & Thomas, G. (2020) 'Coaches' perceptions of decision making in rugby union', *Physical Education and Sport Pedagogy*, 25(4): 394–409.

Mosston, M., & Ashworth, S. (2008) *Teaching Physical Education*. First online edition. Pearson Education.

Nacsport (2023) Sports Analysis Evolved, https://www.nacsport.com, accessed 16th August 2023.

NCCDPHP (2000) 'Chart: 2 to 20 years: girls body mass index for age percentiles', https://www.cdc.gov/growthcharts/data/set1clinical/cj41l024.pdf, accessed 29th January 2022.

Nelson, L.J., & Groom, R. (2012) 'The analysis of athletic performance: Some practical and philosophical considerations', *Sport, Education and Society*, 17(5): 687–701. DOI: 10.1080/13573322.2011.552574

Nelson, L.J., Potrac, P., & Groom, R. (2014) 'Receiving video-based feedback in elite ice-hockey: a player's perspective', *Sport, Education and Society*, 19(1): 19–40. DOI: 10.1080/13573322.2011.613925

Nicholls, S.B., James, N., Bryant, E., & Wells, J. (2018) 'Elite coaches' use and engagement with performance analysis within Olympic and Paralympic sport', *International Journal of Performance Analysis in Sport*, 18(5): 764–779. DOI: 10.1080/24748668.2018.1517290

Nisotaki, M. (2016) 'Trend analysis: addressing opposition quality using regression analysis', M.Sc Dissertation, Cardiff, UK: Cardiff Metropolitan University.

North, J.S., & Williams, M.A. (2019) 'Familiarity detection and pattern perception', In A.M. Williams, & R.C. Jackson (eds.), *Anticipation and decision making in sport* (pp. 23–40). Abingdon, OX; Routledge.

North, J.S., Ward, P., Ericsson., & Williams, A.M. (2011) 'Mechanisms underlying skilled anticipation and recognition in a dynamic and temporally constrained domain', *Memory (Hove)*, 19(2): 155–168. DOI: 10.1080/09658211.2010.541466

O'Connor, D., & Larkin, P. (2015) 'Decision making for rugby', In K. Till, & B. Jones (eds.), *The Science of Sport: Rugby* (pp. 102–112). Wiltshire: Crowood Press.

O'Donoghue, P.G. (2005) 'Normative profiles of sports performance', *International Journal of Performance Analysis of Sport*, 5(1): 104–119. DOI: 10.1080/24748668.2005.11868319

O'Donoghue, P. (2006) 'The use of feedback videos in sport', *International Journal of Performance Analysis in Sport*, 6(2): 1–14 DOI: 10.1080/24748668.2006.11868368

O'Donoghue, P.G. (2009) 'Interacting performances theory', *International Journal of Performance Analysis in Sport*, 9(1): 26–46. DOI: 10.1080/24748668.2009.11868462

O'Donoghue, P.G. (2010) *Research methods in performance analysis of sport*, London: Routledge.

O'Donoghue, P.G. (2015) *An introduction to performance analysis of sport*, London: Routledge.

O'Donoghue, P.G., & Beckley, S. (2023) 'Possession tactics in the UEFA women's EURO 2022 soccer tournament', *International Journal of Performance Analysis in Sport*, 23(1): 48–64. DOI: 10.1080/24748668.2023.2206273

O'Donoghue, P.G., & Holmes, L. (2015) *Data analysis in sport*, London: Routledge.

O'Donoghue, P.G., & Longville, J. (2004) 'Reliability testing and the use of Statistics in performance analysis support: a case study from an international netball tournament', In P.G. O'Donoghue, & M.D. Hughes (eds.), *Performance analysis of sport 6* (pp. 1–7). Cardiff: CPA Press, Cardiff Metropolitan University.

O'Donoghue, P, & Mayes, A. (2013) 'Performance analysis, feedback and communication in coaching', In T. McGarry, P. O'Donoghue, & J. Sampaio (eds.), *Routledge handbook of sports performance analysis* (pp. 155–164). Oxon: Routledge.

O'Donoghue, P.G., Hughes, M.G., Rudkin, S., Bloomfield, J., Cairns, G., & Powell, S. (2005) 'Work-rate analysis using the POWER (Periods of Work Efforts and Recoveries) System', *International Journal of Performance Analysis of Sport*, 5(1): 5–21. DOI: 10.1080/24748668.2005.11868311.

O'Donoghue, P.G., Mayes, A., Edwards, K.M., & Garland, J. (2008) 'Performance norms for British National Super League netball', *International Journal of Sports Science and Coaching*, 3, 501–511. DOI: 10.1260/174795408787186486

O'Donoghue, P., Holmes, L., & Robinson, G. (2017) *Doing a research project in sport performance analysis*, Abingdon: Routledge.

Olsen, E., & Larsen, O. (1997) 'Use of match analysis by coaches', In T. Reilly, J. Bangsbo, & M. Hughes (eds.), *Science and Football III* (pp. 209–220). London: E and FN Spon.

Omoigui, N. (2022) 'The role of data collection in the fight for sporting integrity', https://igamingbusiness.com/social-responsibility/sports-integrity/the-role-of-data-collection-in-the-fight-for-sporting-integrity/, accessed 20th July 2023.

Oriard, M. (2010) *Brand NFL: making and selling America's favourite sport*, University of North Carolina Press.

Palao, J.M., & Morante, J.C. (2013) 'Technical effectiveness', In T. McGarry, P.G. O'Donoghue, & J. Sampaio (eds.), *Routledge handbook of sports performance analysis* (pp. 213–224). Abingdon: Routledge.

Parmar, N. (2023) 'Exciting Middlesex M.Sc Sports Performance Analysis in soccer studentship in collaboration with UEFA', https://twitter.com/NimaiParmar/status/1669362641540640768, accessed 20th July 2023.

Parrington, L., Ball, K., & Macmahon, C. (2013) 'Game-based analysis of handballing in Australian Football', *International Journal of Performance Analysis in Sport*, 13(3): 759–772. DOI: 10.1080/24748668.2013.11868687

Parson, A., Mullen, R., & Hughes, M. (2001) 'Performance profiles of male rugby union players', In M. Hughes, & I.M. Franks (eds.), *Performance analysis, sports science and computing* (pp. 129–137). Cardiff: CPA Press.

Pennington, A. (2014) 'Data drives on-air sports analysis', https://www.thebroadcastbridge.com/content/entry/791/data-drives-on-air-sports-analysis, accessed 19th February 2022.

Pizzera, A., Möller, C., & Plessner, H. (2018) 'Gaze behavior of gymnastics judges: Where do experienced judges and gymnasts look while judging?', *Research Quarterly for Exercise and Sport*, 89(1): 112–119. DOI: 10.1080/02701367.2017.1412392

Poizat, G., Sève, C., & Saury, J. (2013) 'Qualitative aspects of performance analysis', In T., McGarry, P.G. O'Donoghue, & J. Sampaio (eds.), *Routledge handbook of sports performance analysis* (pp. 309–320). London: Routledge.

Prüßner, R., & Siegle, M. (2015) 'Additional time in soccer: influence of league and referee', *International Journal of Performance Analysis in Sport*, 15(2): 551–559. DOI: 10.1080/24748668.2015.11868813

Quinn, R.E., Faerman, S.R., Thompson, M.P., & McGrath, M.R. (1996) *Becoming a master manager: a competency framework,* 2nd edition, New York: Wiley.

Rahimian, P., & Toka, L. (2022) 'Optical tracking in team sports: A survey on player and ball tracking methods in soccer and other team sports', *Journal of Quantitative Analysis in Sports*, 18(1): 35–57. DOI: 10.1515/jqas-2020-0088

Ramos, A. Coutinho, P., Silva, P., Davids, K., Guimarães, E., & Mesquita, I. (2017) 'Entropy measures reveal collective tactical behaviours in volleyball teams: how variability and regularity in game actions influence competitive rankings and match status', *International Journal of Performance Analysis in Sport*, 17(6): 848–862. DOI: 10.1080/24748668.2017.1405611.

Raven, B.H. (1992) 'A power/interaction model of interpersonal influence. French and Raven thirty years later', *Journal of Social Behaviour and Personality*, 7(2): 217–244. DOI: 10.1111/j.1530-2415.2008.00159.x

Raven, B.H., Schwarzwald, J., & Koslowsky, M. (1998) 'Conceptualising and measuring a power/interaction model of interpersonal influence', *Journal of Applied Social Psychology*, 28(4): 307–332. DOI: 10.1111/j.1559-1816.1998.tb01708.x

Raya-Castellano, P.E., & Uriondo, L.F. (2015) 'A review of the multidisciplinary approach to develop elite players at professional football academies: applying science to a professional context', *International Journal of Performance Analysis in Sport*, 15(1): 1–19. DOI: 10.1080/24748668.2015.11868773.

Raya-Castellano, P.E., Reeves, M.J., Littlewood, M., & McRobert, A.P. (2020) 'An exploratory investigation of junior-elite football coaches′ behaviours during video-based feedback sessions', *International Journal of Performance Analysis in Sport*, 20(4): 729–746. DOI: 10.1080/24748668.2020.1782717

Rayner, R., Young, W.B., & Talpey, S.W. (2022) 'The agility demands of Australian football: a notational analysis', *International Journal of Performance Analysis in Sport*, 22(4): 621–637. DOI: 10.1080/24748668.2022.2106112

Redwood-Brown, A.J., O'Donoghue, P.G., Nevill, A.M., Saward, C., & Sunderland, C. (2019) 'Effects of playing position, pitch location, opposition ability and team ability on the technical performance of elite soccer players in different score line states', *PLoS ONE*, 14(2): e0211707, DOI: 10.1371/journal.pone.0211707

Reilly, T., & Thomas, V. (1976) 'A motion analysis of work rate in different positional roles in professional football match play', *Journal of Human Movement Studies*, 2, 87–97.

Robertson, S.P. (2020) 'Man and machine: adaptive tools for the contemporary performance analyst', *Journal of Sports Sciences*, 38(18): 2118–2126. DOI: 10.1080/02640414.2020.1774143

Roldán-Márquez, R., Onetti-Onetti, W., Alvero-Cruz, J.R., & Castillo-Rodríguez, A. (2022) 'Win or lose. Physical and physiological responses in paddle tennis competition according to the game result', *International Journal of Performance Analysis in Sport*, 22(4): 479–490. DOI: 10.1080/24748668.2022.2082173

Røsseland, A. (2018) 'The effect of video telestration on pattern recognition and postural cue usage in elite football', Unpublished M.Sc thesis, University of Chester.

SantAnna, R.T., Roberts, S.P., Moore, L.J., & Stokes, K.A. (2021) 'Referee positioning, but not match demands, score difference, or field location, are associated with breakdown decision-making accuracy in elite rugby sevens referees', International Journal of Performance Analysis in Sport, 21(6):, 1127–1139. DOI: 10.1080/24748668.2021.1979824

Sarmento, H., Anguera, M.T., Pereira, A., Marques, A., Campaniço, J., & Leitão, J. (2014) 'Patterns of play in the counterattack of elite football teams: a mixed method approach', *International Journal of Performance Analysis in Sport*, 14(2): 411–427. DOI: 10.1080/24748668.2014.11868731

Schmucker, C., Schell, L.K., Portalupi, S., Oeller, P., Cabrera, L., Bassler, D., Schwarzer, G., Scherer, R.W., Antes, G., von Elm, E., & Meerpohl, J.J. (2023) 'OPEN consortium. Extent of non-publication in cohorts of studies approved by research ethics committees or included in trial registries', *PLoS One*, 9(12): e114023. DOI: 10.1371/journal.pone.0114023

Sedano, S., Vaeyens, R., Philippaerts, R.M., Redondo, J.C., & Cuadrado, G. (2009) 'Anthropometric and anaerobic fitness profile of elite and non-elite female soccer players', *Journal of Sports Medicine and Physical Fitness*, 49: 387–394, PMID: 20087298

Shore, E.G. (1971) 'Analysis of a multi-institutional series of completed cases', Presentation at the Scientific Integrity Symposium, Harvard Medical School, Boston (cited in Thomas and Nelson, 1996: 74–78).

Slate (2018) 'Football's Magic Crayon', https://www.youtube.com/watch?v=_5Tw4zm0fNs, accessed: 1st December 2022.

Smeeton, N.J., Hüttermann, S., & Williams, M.A. (2019) 'Postural cues, biological motion perception, and anticipation on sport', In A.M. Williams, & R.C. Jackson (eds.), *Anticipation and decision making in sport* (pp. 1–22). Abingdon, Oxon; Routledge.

Smith, J., Rands, S., Bateman, M., & Francis, J. (2022) 'Assessing the efficacy of video telestration in aiding memory recall among elite professional football players', *Sports Innovation Journal*, 1: 61–81. DOI: 10.18060/26317

StatsPerform (2022) 'Opta data from StatsPerform', https://www.statsperform.com/opta/, accessed 29th January 2022.

Tenga, A.P.C., Holme, I., Ronglan, L.T., & Bahr, R. (2010) 'Effect of match location on playing tactics for goal scoring in Norwegian professional soccer', *Journal of Sport Behaviour,* 33, 89–108. DOI: 10.1080/02640410903502774

Thomas, J.R., & Nelson, J.K. (1996) *Research methods in physical activity,* Champaign, IL: Human Kinetics.

Thomas, G. (2007) 'Real-time camera tracking using sports pitch markings', *Journal of Real-Time Image Processing,* 2: 2–3. DOI: 10.1007/s11554-007-0041-1

Thomas, G., & Edwards, C. (2022) 'Developing football coaching practice to improve players' tactical flexibility and game intelligence using video analysis', *FIFA Technical Report, Zurich,* Switzerland: FIFA. DOI: 10.13140/RG.2.2.24636.92806

Thomas, G., Gade, R., Moeslund, T., Carr, P., & Hilton, A. (2017) 'Computer vision for sports: current applications and research topics', *Computer Vision and Image Understanding,* 159, 3–18. DOI: 10.1016/j.cviu.2017.04.011

Timmons, K., Collins, K., & Mangan, S. (2022) 'An analysis of the effectiveness of kickouts in sub-elite Gaelic football', *International Journal of Performance Analysis in Sport,* 22(4): 526–540. DOI: 10.1080/24748668.2022.2086515

UK Sports Institute (2023) 'Support Services', https://www.uksportsinstitute.co.uk, accessed 16th August 2023.

US Open (2021a) 'IBM Slam Tracker, Women's Singles Final', https://www.usopen.org/en_US/scores/stats/2701.html?promo=matchchanger, accessed 29th January 2022.

US Open (2021b) 'IBM Slam Tracker, Women's Singles Second Round', https://www.usopen.org/en_US/scores/stats/2204.html, accessed 29th January 2022.

US Open (2021c) 'Emma Raducanu vs Shuai Zhang Highlights: 2021 US Open Round 2', https://www.youtube.com/watch?v=OqgZnHhDZO0, accessed 29th January 2022.

Van Haaren, J., Robberechts, P., Decroos, T., Bransen, L., Davis, J., Ric, A., & Peláez, R. (2019) 'Analysing performance and playing style using ball event data', In Á. Ric, & R. Peláez (eds.), *Football Analytics: Now and Beyond. A deep dive into the current state of advanced data analytics* (pp. 36–47). Barcelona, Spain: Barça Innovation Hub.

Vandewalle, D., Gilbert, P., & Monod, H. (1987) 'Standard anaerobic tests', *Sports Medicine,* 4(4): 268–289. DOI: 10.2165/00007256-198704040-00004

Vargha, A., & Delaney, H.D. (2000) 'A critique and improvement of the CL common language effect size statistics of McGraw and Wong', *Journal of Educational and Behavioral Statistics,* 25(2):101–132. DOI: 10.3102/10769986025002101

Vítor de Assis, J., González-Víllora, S., Clemente, F.M., Cardoso, F., & Teoldo, I. (2020) 'Do youth soccer players with different tactical behaviour also perform differently in decision-making and visual search strategies?', *International Journal of Performance Analysis in Sport,* 20(6): 1143–1156. DOI: 10.1080/24748668.2020.1838784

Vivian, R., Mullen, R., & Hughes, M. (2001) 'Performance profiles at league, European Cup and International levels of male rugby union players, with specific reference to flankers, number 8s and number 9s', In M.D. Hughes, & I. Franks (eds.), *Fifth world congress of performance analysis of sport* (pp. 137–143). Cardiff: CPA Press, Cardiff Metropolitan University.

Whoscored (2023) 'Premier league referee statistics', https://www.whoscored.com/Regions/252/Tournaments/2/Seasons/9075/Stages/20934/RefereeStatistics/England-Premier-League-2022-2023, accessed 20th July 2023.

Williams, J.J. (2012) 'Operational definitions in performance analysis and the need for consensus', *International Journal of Performance Analysis of Sport*, 12: 52–63. DOI: 10.1080/24748668.2012.11868582

Williams, A.M., & Jackson., R.C. (2019) *Anticipation and decision making in sport*, Abingdon, OX: Routledge.

Wiltshire, H.D. (2013) 'Sports performance analysis for high performance managers', In T. McGarry, P.G. O'Donoghue, & J. Sampaio (eds.), *Routledge handbook of sports performance analysis* (pp. 176–186). London: Routledge.

Wimbledon (2023) Wimbledon IBM SlamTracker, https://www.wimbledon.com, accessed 14th August 2023.

Wixted, J.T., & Wells, G.L. (2017) 'The relationship between eyewitness confidence and identification accuracy: a new synthesis', *Psychological Science in the Public Interest*, 18: 10–16. DOI: 10.1177/1529100616686966

Wright, C., Atkins, S., & Jones, B. (2012) 'An analysis of elite coaches' engagement with performance analysis services (match, notational analysis and technique analysis)', *International Journal of Performance Analysis in Sport*, 12(2): 436–451. DOI: 10.1080/24748668.2012.11868609

Wright, C., Carling, C., & Collins, D. (2014) 'The wider context of performance analysis and its application in the football coaching process', *International Journal of Performance Analysis in Sport*, 14(3): 709–733. DOI: 10.1080/24748668.2014.11868753

Wright, C., Carling, C., Lawlor, C., & Collins, D. (2016) 'Elite football player engagement with performance analysis', *International Journal of Performance Analysis in Sport*, 16(3): 1007–1032. DOI: 10.1080/24748668.2016.11868945.

Index